THE EASY AND TASTY DASH DIET COOKBOOK FOR SENIORS

Nourish Your Body With Full-Color Low-Sodium Recipes Designed to Lower Blood Pressure, Boost Heart Health, and Support Healthy Aging After 60, With a 30-Day Meal Plan to Guide Your Journey.

Amber Hampton

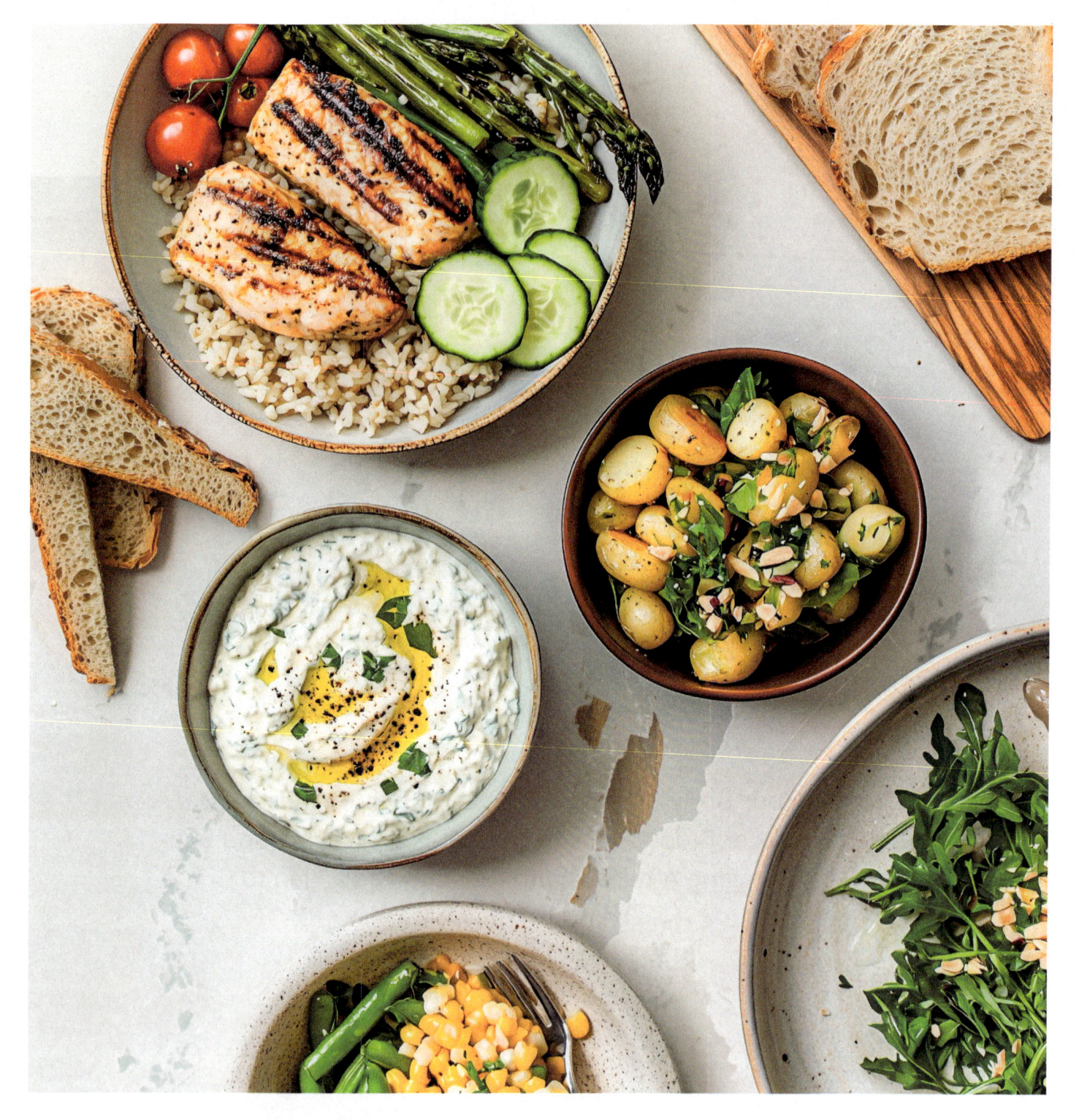

© COPYRIGHT 2025 – AMBER HAMPTON & BALANCED LIVING BOOKS – ALL RIGHTS RESERVED.

The content contained within this book may not be reproduced, duplicated or transmitted without direct written permission from the author or the publisher.

Under no circumstances will any blame or legal responsibility be held against the publisher or author for any damages, reparation, or monetary loss due to the information contained within this book, either directly or indirectly.

Legal Notice:

This book is copyright protected. It is only for personal use. You cannot amend, distribute, sell, use, quote, or paraphrase any part of the content within this book without the consent of the author or publisher.

Disclaimer Notice:

Please note the information contained within this document is for educational and informational purposes only. While every effort has been made to ensure accuracy and clarity, this book is not a substitute for professional medical advice. Always consult your dietitian or healthcare provider before making any significant changes to your diet or lifestyle. The author and publisher disclaim any responsibility for any adverse effects resulting directly or indirectly from the information presented in this book.

By reading this document, the reader agrees that under no circumstances is the author responsible for any loss, damage, or injury, direct or indirect, that may occur as a result of the use or misuse of the information contained herein.

TABLE OF CONTENTS

BONUS RESOURCES — 6
INTRODUCTION — 8

CHAPTER 1 – THE DASH DIET ESSENTIALS — 10
- What Is the DASH Diet, Really? — 10
- Why It Works: The Science Made Simple — 10
- Common Myths and Misconceptions — 11
- Why It's Perfect for Seniors — 11

CHAPTER 2 – DASH MADE EASY — 12
- A Practical Guide for Everyday Life — 12
- The DASH Plate: A Visual Guide to Meals — 12
- How Much Should You Eat? — 13
- Understanding Daily Portions — 13
- The Key to Balance: Sodium & Smart Choices — 14

CHAPTER 3 – YOUR 30-DAY DASH MEAL PLAN — 16
- Before You Begin: What You'll Need — 16
- The 30 Day Plan — 16
- Before You Cook — 19

CHAPTER 4 – DASH RECIPES MADE FOR YOU

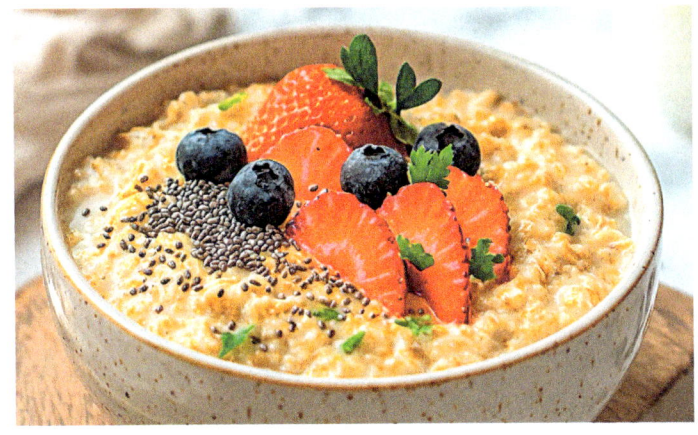

BREAKFAST — 21
- Creamy Oatmeal with Berries — 22
- Frittata with Spinach & Mushrooms — 22
- Greek Yogurt Parfait with Homemade Granola — 23
- Warm Veggie Breakfast Burrito — 23
- Mini Banana Oat Loaf — 24
- Cottage Cheese Bowl with Caramelized Peach — 24
- Soft-Baked Blueberry Oat Bars — 25
- Savory Sweet Potato & Broccoli Hash — 25
- Fluffy Whole Wheat Banana Pancakes — 26
- Spinach & Tomato Morning Scramble — 26
- Apple Cinnamon Muffins with a DASH Twist — 27
- Pumpkin Hazelnut Breakfast Loaf — 27
- Avocado & Egg Breakfast Toast with Lemon & Dill — 28
- Tropical Mango & Coconut Smoothie Bowl — 28
- Savory Black Bean & Avocado Morning Wrap — 29
- Golden Toast with Ricotta & Pear Delight — 29
- Hearty Seeded Whole Grain Bread — 30
- Easy Olive & Herb Bread — 30

LUNCH — 31
- Zesty Grilled Chicken & Rice Salad — 32
- Mediterranean Chickpea Power Bowl — 32
- Hearty Lentil & Veggie Soup — 33
- Stuffed Sweet Potato with Black Beans & Avocado — 33
- Butternut Squash Cream with Homemade Croutons — 34
- Oven-Baked Stuffed Bell Peppers — 34
- Comforting Chicken Noodle Soup — 35

CONTENTS

- Salmon Cakes with Sautéed Kale — 35
- Zucchini Noodles with homemade DASH Pesto — 36
- Colorful Shrimp & Avocado Bowl — 36
- Savory Turkey & Veggie Lettuce Wraps — 37
- Chickpea & Spinach Wraps with Creamy Yogurt Sauce — 37
- Stuffed Turkey Meatballs with Spinach & Tomato — 38
- Whole Wheat Pasta with Sautéed Veggies — 38
- Shakshuka with Spinach & Bell Peppers — 39
- Creamy Lemon Fettuccine with Shrimp — 39
- Curried Cauliflower Steaks with Red Rice & Tzatziki — 40
- Salmon & Couscous Salad with Fresh Greens — 40

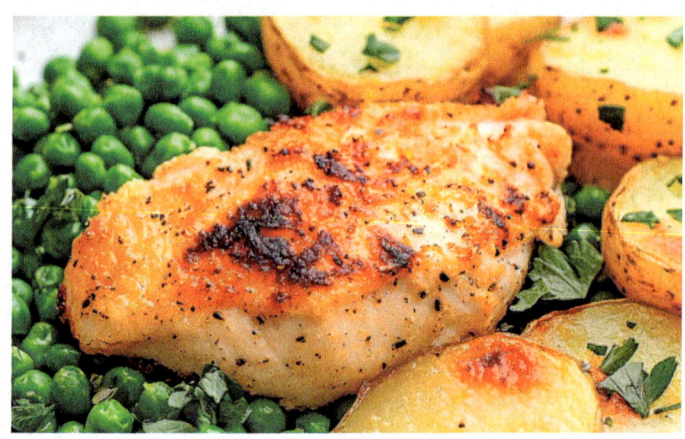

DINNER — 41

- Lemon & Garlic Chicken with Sautéed Veggies — 42
- Spiced Lentil Patties with Fresh Salad — 42
- Fresh Fish with Colorful Veggie Medley — 43
- Eggplants with Tasty Lentils & Mushrooms — 43
- Shrimp Stir-Fry with Colorful Veggies — 44
- Healthy Turkey & Spinach Lasagna — 44
- Salmon with Herbed Yogurt & Roasted Veggies — 45
- Light Tropical Chicken Curry — 45
- Tender Herb-Crusted Pork with Garden Veggies — 46
- Hake en Papillote with Lemon, Zucchini & Eggplant — 46
- Baked Chicken with Apple & Mashed Cauliflower — 47
- Warm & Rustic Beef Stew — 47
- Gentle Cod Curry with Veggies — 48
- Pork Tenderloin with Fennel Sauce — 48
- Cozy White Bean Stew with a Twist — 49
- Tilapia with Fresh Garden Salad & Lemon Vinaigrette — 49
- Mediterranean Chicken with Orzo & Veggies — 50
- Asian-Style Ginger Tofu & Veggie Stir-Fry — 50

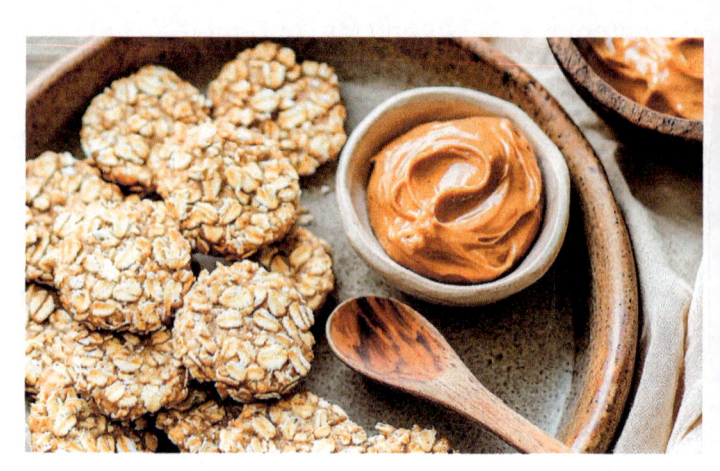

SNACKS & DRINKS — 51

- No-Bake Oat Bites with Peanut Butter & Seeds — 52
- Creamy Hummus with Roasted Veggie Sticks — 52
- DASH Tzatziki Sauce — 53
- Sweet Baked Apple Slices with a Nutty Twist — 53
- Creamy Avocado & White Bean Dip — 54
- Spicy Dash Trail Mix — 54
- Mini Baked Lentil Falafels with Yogurt-Herb Dip — 55
- Sweet Potato Toasts with Cottage Cheese & Walnuts — 55
- Crunchy Seed Crackers with Herbs — 56
- Citrusy DASH Guacamole — 56
- DASH-Friendly Popcorn — 57
- Savory Roll-Ups with Turkey, Avocado & Spinach — 57
- Homemade Baked Veggie Chips — 58
- Green Revitalizing Smoothie — 58
- Berry Yogurt Shake with a Twist — 59
- Piña Colada DASH-Friendly Mocktail — 59
- Red Antioxidant Smoothie — 60
- Pumpkin Pie Smoothie — 60

DESSERTS — 61

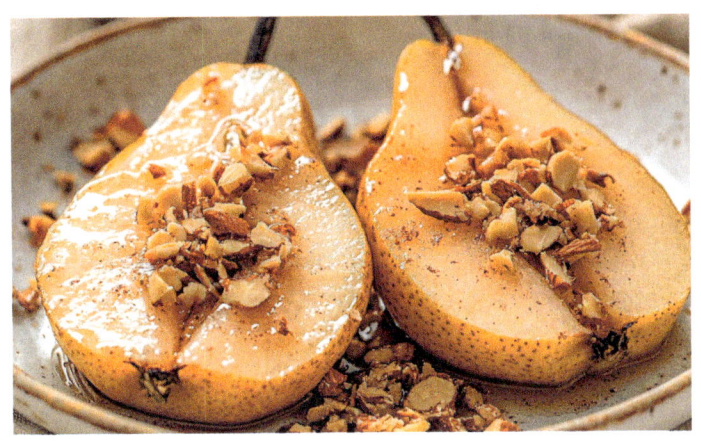

- Warm Cinnamon-Baked Pears — 62
- Zesty Lemon Yogurt Mousse — 62
- Chocolate-Dipped Fruit Skewers — 63
- Tiramisu in a Cup — 63
- Mini Carrot & Walnut Cakes — 64
- Creamy DASH Cheesecake — 64
- Chocolate Pistachio Oat Cookies — 65
- Chia & Mango Pudding — 65
- Cocoa & Walnut Mug Cake — 66
- Rhubarb & Pecan Muffins — 66
- American-Style Apple Crumble — 67
- Light Chocolate Pudding — 67
- Mediterranean Baked Apricots with a Twist — 68
- Warm Berry Crisp with Oat Topping — 68

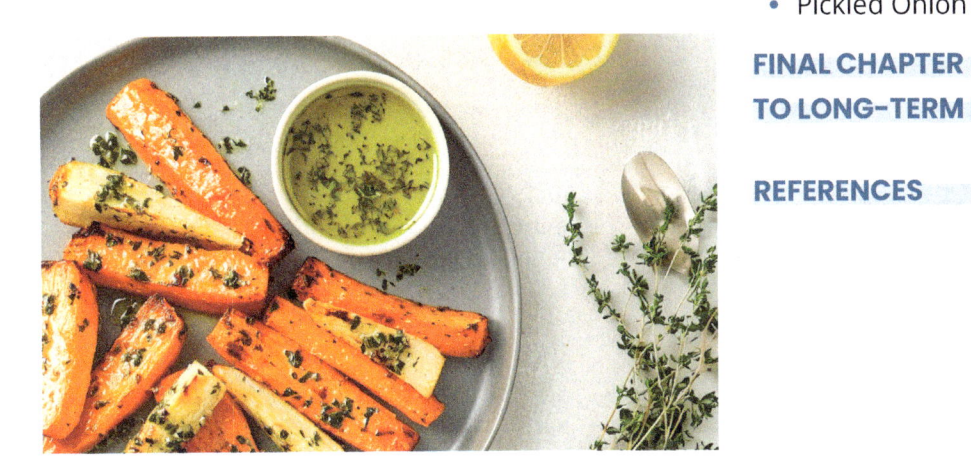

SIDES & EXTRAS — 69

- Mini Egg Muffins with Spinach & Tomato — 70
- Rainbow Coleslaw with Light Dressing — 70
- Mediterranean Eggplant Dip (Baba Ganoush) — 71
- Green Beans with Toasted Almonds — 71
- Mediterranean Tomato & Tuna Bites — 72
- Roasted Butternut Squash with a Twist — 72
- Sautéed Kale with Cherry Tomatoes — 73
- Nourishing Couscous with Mushrooms & Swiss Chard — 73
- Simple Ratatouille Bake — 74
- Basil-Ginger Stuffed Mushrooms — 74
- Roasted Carrot & Parsnip Wedges with Thyme — 75
- Balsamic Roasted Brussels Sprouts with Walnuts — 75
- Creamy Tuna Spread — 76
- Pickled Onion & Carrot Slaw — 76

FINAL CHAPTER – YOUR PATH TO LONG-TERM HEALT — 78

REFERENCES — 80

BONUS RESOURCES FOR LIVING THE DASH WAY

Before anything else, I'd like to thank you for choosing this cookbook and inviting me into your kitchen.

As a token of my appreciation, I've created some additional resources to support your journey toward better health.

Making lasting changes can be challenging—but having the right tools can make all the difference. That's why I've created a set of exclusive, free resources that complement the content of this book and help you stay confident, supported, and motivated every step of the way:

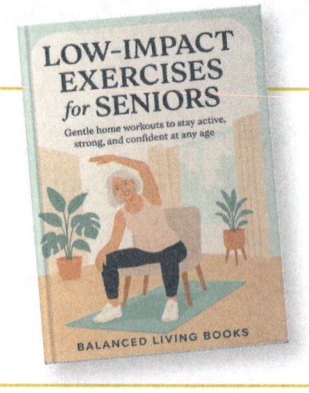

Low-Impact Exercises for Seniors

Gentle and effective routines to help you feel more energized and move with ease every day.

This ebook is perfect for older adults who want to stay active, strong, and confident—from the comfort of home.

DASH Dining Delights: Special Occasion Recipes

Heart-healthy recipes designed for holidays, celebrations, and meaningful moments.

These festive DASH-adapted meals let you enjoy special occasions while supporting your health goals.

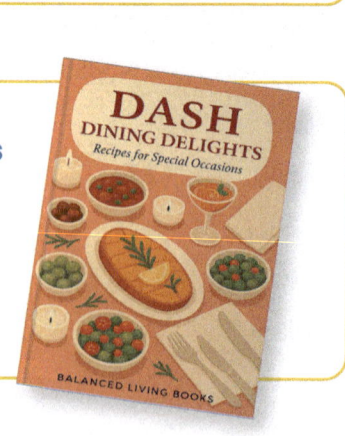

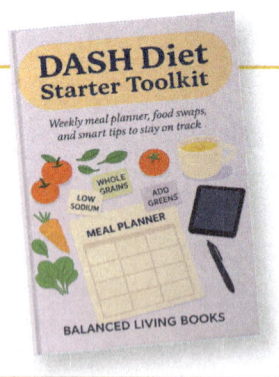

DASH Diet Starter Toolkit

Weekly meal planner, food swaps, and smart tips to stay on track.

Designed to simplify your routine, support your planning, and boost confident, balanced choices every day

TO ACCESS THESE FREE RESOURCES, SIMPLY SCAN THE QR CODE

If you prefer, you can also download them directly at: https://balancedlivingbooks.com/dash-gift/

Or, you can email us at info@balancedlivingbooks.com with the magic word "**DASHDIETGIFT**" and I'll personally send them straight to your inbox.

If you have any questions, suggestions, or feedback about this cookbook, just send me an email—I'm here to help!

I recommend bookmarking this page for easy reference. As you continue exploring this cookbook, you'll find these free resources especially helpful for putting the DASH principles into practice.

Thank you for trusting me on this journey. Now, let's keep moving forward—together.

A LITTLE ABOUT ME

Before we dive into the heart of this book, I'd love to take a moment to introduce myself—so you can know a little more about the person behind these pages.

Cooking and eating well have always been close to my heart—not just as habits, but as acts of care.

Over the years, I've dedicated myself to helping older adults discover a way of eating that feels joyful, simple, and sustainable—not complicated or restrictive.

Through my books, I focus on creating practical tools that support real lives: easy, flavorful recipes grounded in the best nutrition principles for heart health and overall well-being.

I believe that good food should nourish both your body and your spirit. And it should be something you look forward to, not something you have to endure.

Each page I create, each recipe I share, is built with one clear mission: to help you feel more confident, more energized, and more at peace with the way you care for yourself.

Thank you for trusting me to be part of your journey.

Here's to many more moments of joy, connection, and heart-healthy living.

Amber Hampton

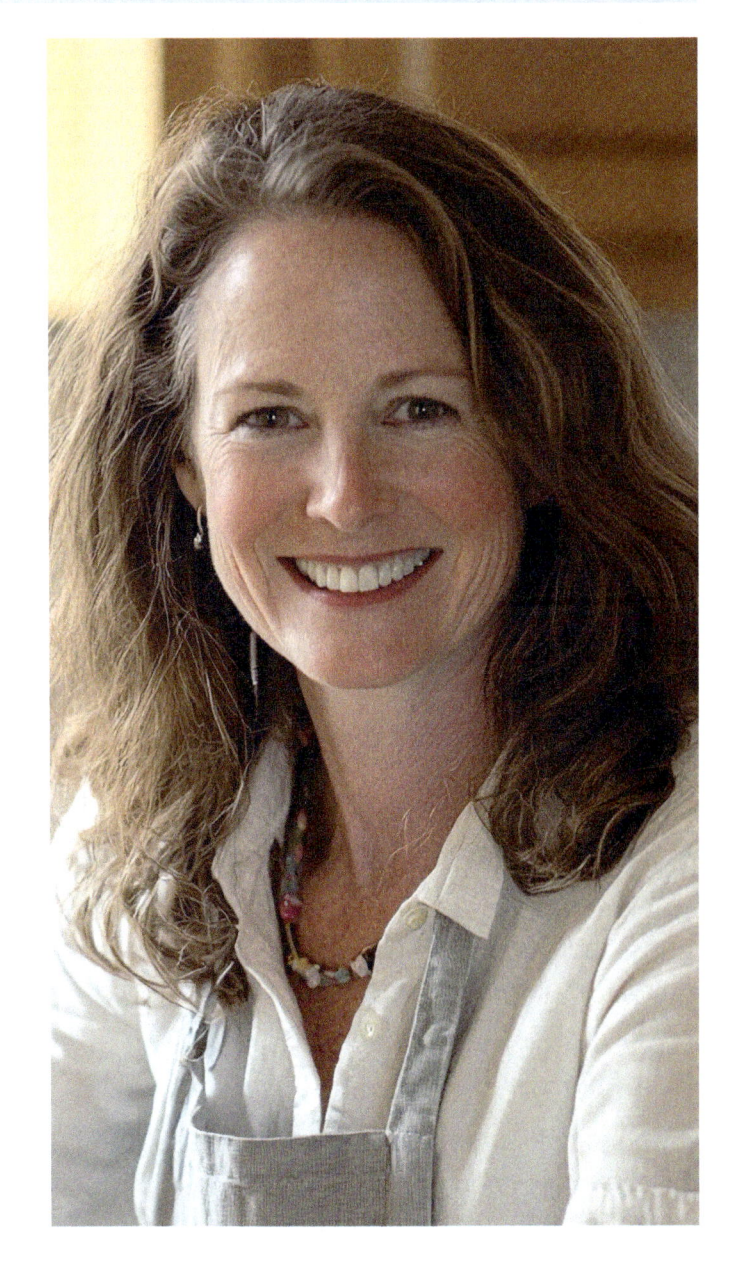

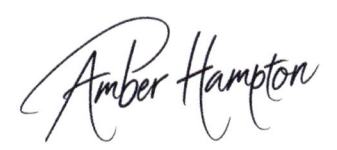

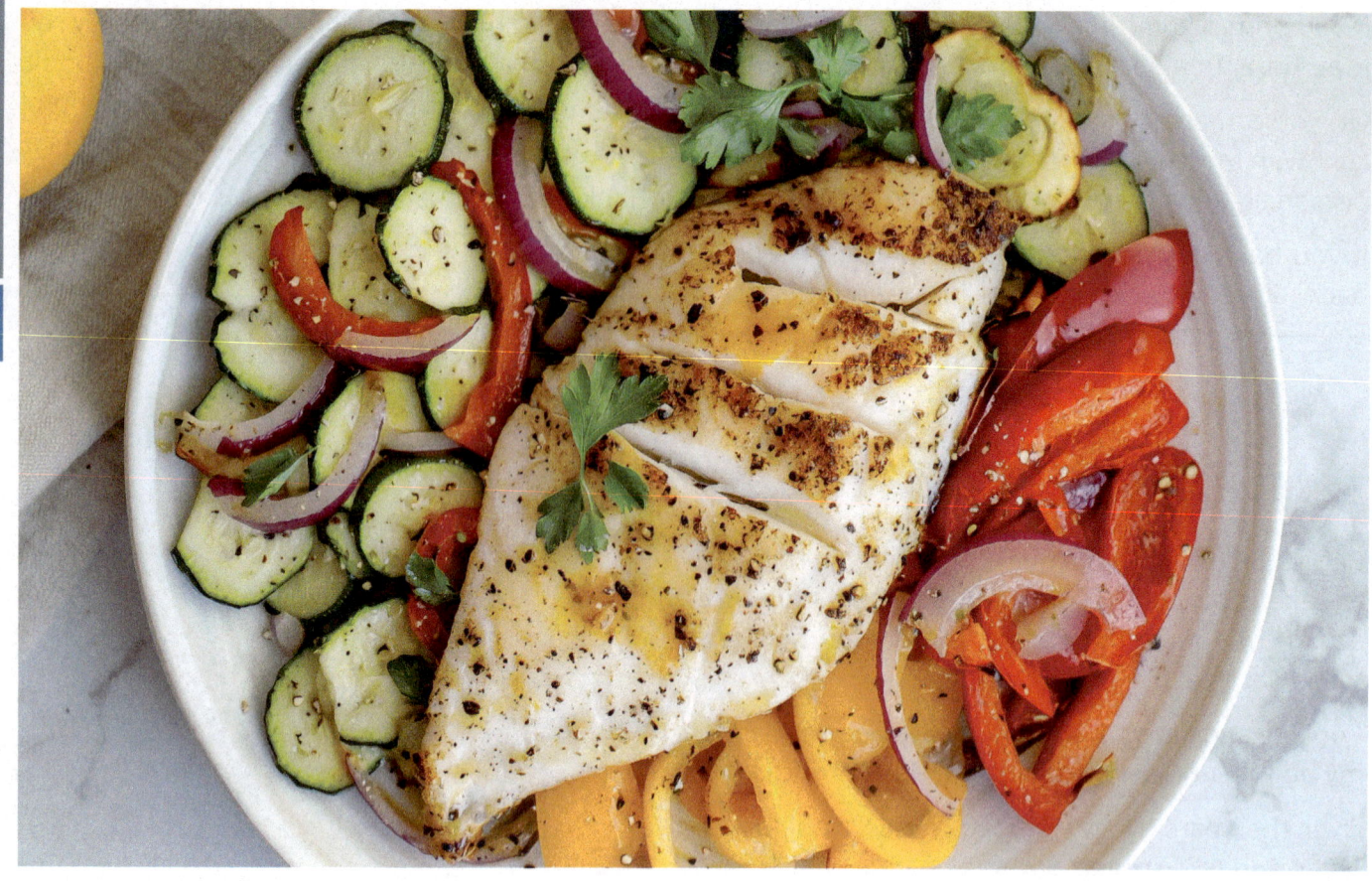

INTRODUCTION

What if taking care of your health didn't mean giving up the joy of eating well?

What if, instead of counting calories or cutting out everything you love, you could lower your blood pressure while enjoying every bite?

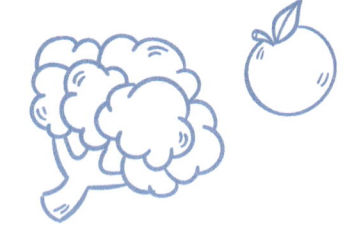

At 69, Helen had already tried everything.

She had been prescribed blood pressure medications, and she'd tried cutting out salt, bread—even dairy. But nothing seemed to work.

Every doctor's visit ended the same way: more frustration... and another pill.

Helen didn't want another diet. She wanted a solution she could stick to. Something that made sense. Something that fit her pace, her age, and her kitchen.

That was one of the first conversations I had with a reader like you. And it changed the way I decided to write this book.

Because the truth is that eating well doesn't have to feel like a punishment.

You shouldn't be afraid to open the fridge. Cooking something healthy shouldn't feel impossible or bland.

Many of my readers come to this point feeling confused, frustrated, or simply exhausted by all the conflicting information out there.

They want to take care of their heart, lower their blood pressure, or reduce cholesterol—but without giving up the joy of food, of cooking something tasty for their grandkids, or sharing a guilt-free dinner.

And that's where the DASH diet comes in.

Not as a trend. Not as a list of restrictions.

DASH is a realistic, flexible, and science-backed lifestyle, designed to help you improve your health without stress, calorie counting, or boring meals.

This book isn't a list of "don'ts" or just another strict diet.

It's a practical guide made for people who want to eat better without the overwhelm, rediscover the joy of food, and take better care of their heart in the process.

Whether you've been advised to try the DASH diet due to high blood pressure or cholesterol, or you simply want to feel more energized and vibrant again—you're in the right place.

Here, you'll find real tools to help you do just that:

A complete 30-Day meal plan, weekly shopping lists, easy and flavorful recipes, and senior-friendly tips tailored to your lifestyle.

My goal isn't just to help you eat better.

I want you to feel better. To regain energy, motivation, and joy every time you sit down at the table. To have a guide you can rely on—no extremes, no confusion.

- ✓ **THIS BOOK IS YOURS. THIS PATH IS YOURS.**
- ✓ **AND I'M HERE TO WALK IT WITH YOU, ONE RECIPE AT A TIME, ONE DAY AT A TIME.**
- ✓ **BECAUSE IT'S NEVER TOO LATE TO TAKE CARE OF YOUR HEART.**
- ✓ **AND IT'S NEVER TOO LATE TO FALL IN LOVE WITH FOOD AGAIN.**

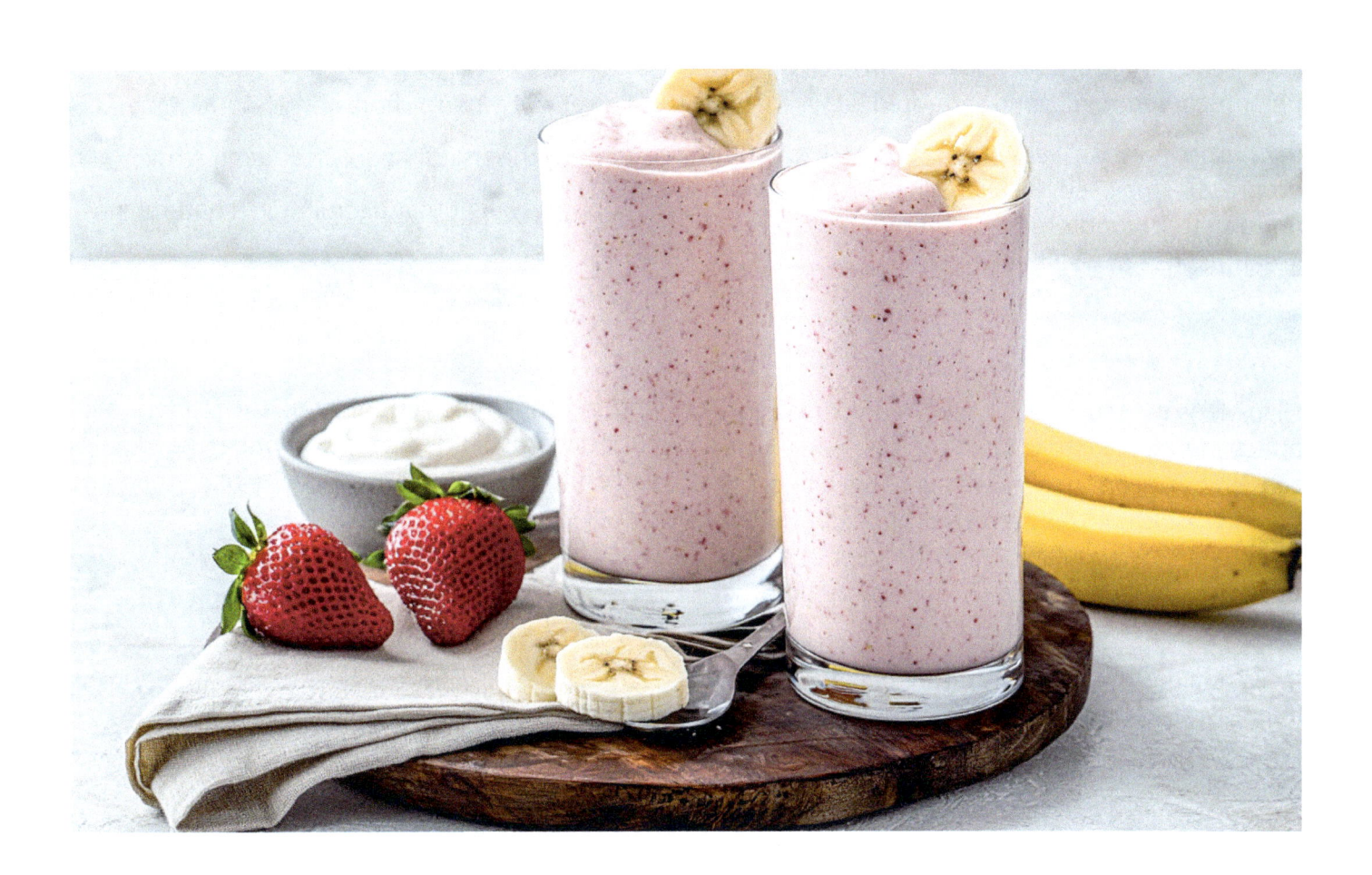

CHAPTER 1: THE DASH DIET ESSENTIALS

1.1 WHAT IS THE DASH DIET, REALLY?

If you've ever been told by your doctor to "watch your salt," you're not alone. That simple advice has led millions of people to discover the DASH diet—short for Dietary Approaches to Stop Hypertension. But let's be clear: DASH isn't another fad or temporary food trend. It's a practical, long-term approach to eating that supports your heart, your blood pressure, and your overall health.

Originally developed by researchers and medical professionals to combat high blood pressure, the DASH diet has been consistently recommended by the National Institutes of Health, the American Heart Association, and countless physicians. Its goal? To help you eat in a way that supports your body—especially as you age—without eliminating joy or flavor from your plate.

Unlike restrictive diets, DASH focuses on balance and nourishment. It emphasizes foods you probably already enjoy: fresh vegetables, fruits, whole grains, lean proteins, and low-fat dairy. And instead of handing you a list of forbidden items, it gently encourages you to cut back on excess sodium, processed foods, and saturated fats.

In short, DASH isn't about perfection. It's about progress—small, sustainable changes that add up to better blood pressure, more energy, and a greater sense of well-being.

1.2 WHY IT WORKS: THE SCIENCE MADE SIMPLE

High blood pressure (also known as hypertension) affects nearly 1 in 2 adults in the U.S.—and it becomes more common as we age. That's because blood vessels naturally stiffen over time, and lifestyle habits accumulate. The DASH diet works by targeting the root causes of elevated blood pressure, not just masking the symptoms.

How? Mainly through a smarter balance of key minerals your body needs: less sodium and more potassium, magnesium, and calcium—all naturally found in fresh, whole foods.

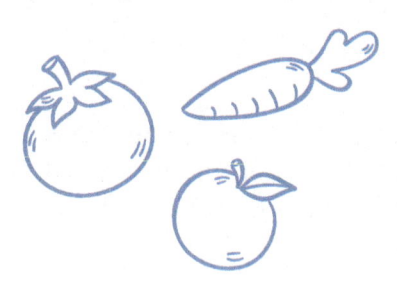

Here's what happens when you eat DASH-style:

- Your body retains less water and bloating decreases
- Your blood vessels relax and expand more easily
- Your heart doesn't have to work as hard to pump blood
- Over time, this can reduce your blood pressure significantly—often as much as medication

But beyond blood pressure, DASH also helps:

- Lower LDL ("bad") cholesterol
- Reduce the risk of heart attack and stroke
- Support weight management in a natural, no-fuss way
- Improve energy, sleep, digestion, and even mood

And perhaps most importantly for readers over 60: it does all of this gently, without extreme rules or restrictions. That's why DASH has stood the test of time.

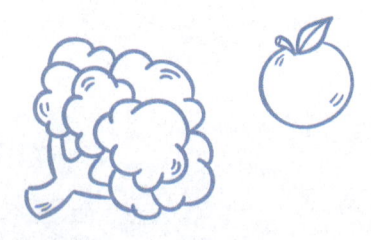

1.3 COMMON MYTHS AND MISCONCEPTIONS

Let's clear a few things up before we go any further.

> **Myth #1:** "The DASH diet is only for people with high blood pressure."
>
> ✓ **Reality:** DASH was designed for heart health, but its benefits go far beyond that. Many people follow it to manage weight, improve cholesterol, reduce fatigue, or simply feel better overall.
>
> **Myth #2:** "It's boring or too bland."
>
> ✓ **Reality:** Not at all. DASH encourages real food—colorful, flavorful, and varied. In this book, you'll find delicious recipes like lemon herb salmon, spiced lentil soup, or banana oat pancakes. Nothing boring here!
>
> **Myth #3:** "It's too hard to follow or too expensive."
>
> ✓ **Reality:** You don't need fancy ingredients or complicated plans. This book is filled with simple meals using affordable, easy-to-find items—many of which you probably already have in your kitchen.
>
> Starting DASH doesn't require an overhaul of your life. It just takes a willingness to begin, one step (or one recipe) at a time.

1.4 WHY IT'S PERFECT FOR SENIORS

As we age, our nutritional needs shift. The body becomes more sensitive to sodium, less efficient at absorbing certain nutrients, and often a bit slower to digest heavy or processed foods. That's where DASH shines.

It's a gentle, heart-smart way of eating that aligns beautifully with the needs of seniors. It supports:

- **Blood pressure regulation** without extremes
- **Bone health** thanks to increased calcium and magnesium
- **Improved digestion** due to higher fiber intake
- **Stable energy levels** through balanced carbs and proteins
- **Mental clarity and mood** by reducing inflammatory foods

What's more, DASH meals are easy to adapt. Whether you're cooking for yourself, your partner, or a family gathering, the recipes in this book are flexible, satisfying, and don't require hours in the kitchen.

It's never too late to feel better. And DASH isn't a reset—it's a new rhythm.

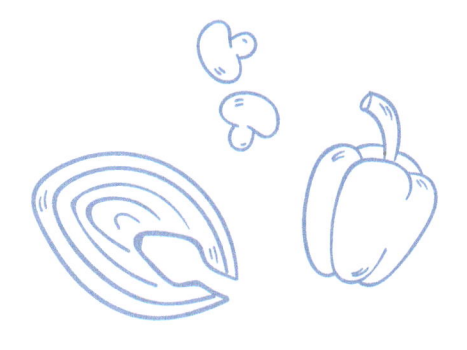

CHAPTER 2: DASH MADE EASY

2.1 A PRACTICAL GUIDE FOR EVERYDAY LIFE

You already know that eating better can change your health. But how do you actually do it—without turning your life upside down?

Eating well doesn't have to be complicated. With DASH, the key is balance—on your plate, in your day, and in your life. That means choosing the right foods in the right amounts without overthinking every bite.

Instead of counting calories or cutting out entire food groups, DASH focuses on adding more of what truly nourishes you: fresh vegetables, whole grains, lean proteins, and heart-healthy fats. It's not about restriction—it's about abundance.

It all starts with how you build a meal. A simple plate can tell you everything you need to know: what to eat more of, what to limit, and how to feel satisfied and energized without going overboard.

But before we talk about portions or meal structure, let's get to know the building blocks of the DASH lifestyle.

These six food groups are the foundation of the DASH diet. Getting familiar with them will help you make quick, confident choices in your daily meals.

2.2 THE DASH PLATE: A VISUAL GUIDE TO MEALS

Now that you know the six essential food groups, it's time to bring them together on your plate.

The DASH Plate is a simple visual tool designed to help you eat in balance. It's a clear and easy way to see how to nourish your body at each meal.

Here's the idea: Divide your plate like this:

- **½ vegetables and/or fruits:** These provide vitamins, minerals, fiber, and antioxidants. Think roasted carrots, spinach salad, sautéed zucchini, apple slices, or orange segments.

- **¼ whole grains:** This could be brown rice, whole wheat pasta, oats, quinoa, or a slice of whole grain bread.

- **¼ lean protein:** Like grilled chicken, baked fish, lentils, tofu, or a couple of boiled eggs.

- **On the side:** A source of low-fat dairy. Such as a small glass of milk, a bit of low-fat yogurt, or cottage cheese.

- **And don't forget healthy fats:** A drizzle of olive oil, a few avocado slices, or a sprinkle of unsalted nuts can make your meal more satisfying and support heart health.

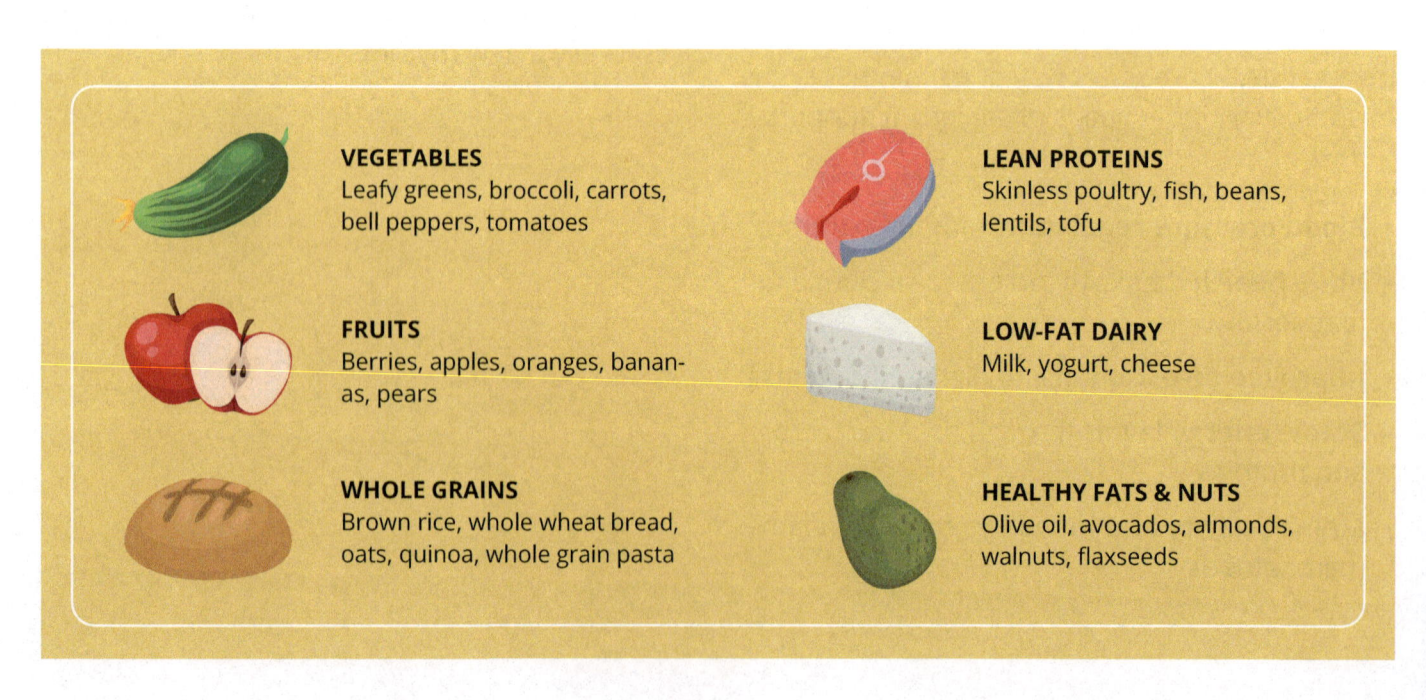

VEGETABLES
Leafy greens, broccoli, carrots, bell peppers, tomatoes

FRUITS
Berries, apples, oranges, bananas, pears

WHOLE GRAINS
Brown rice, whole wheat bread, oats, quinoa, whole grain pasta

LEAN PROTEINS
Skinless poultry, fish, beans, lentils, tofu

LOW-FAT DAIRY
Milk, yogurt, cheese

HEALTHY FATS & NUTS
Olive oil, avocados, almonds, walnuts, flaxseeds

The DASH Plate

½ Vegetables
¼ Whole grains
¼ Lean protein

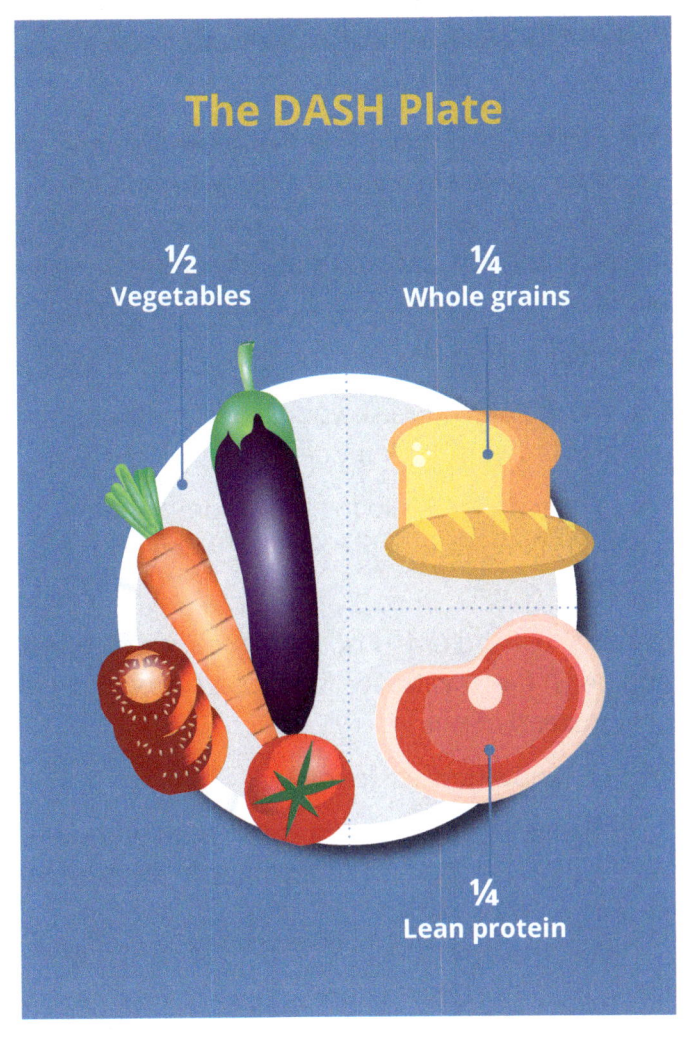

> **Expert Tip:** "Start with the vegetables first when building your plate. It helps fill you up and keeps portions of grains and protein in check."

2.3 HOW MUCH SHOULD YOU EAT? UNDERSTANDING DAILY PORTIONS

One of the strengths of the DASH diet is that it doesn't require counting calories or weighing every bite. Instead, it focuses on daily servings from each food group. A simple, flexible approach that lets you eat intuitively, while still supporting your heart and overall health.

But what exactly is a "serving"? In DASH, it refers to a standard portion of food, based on nutritional value—not the amount you happen to put on your plate. Once you know how many servings you should aim for in a day, building meals becomes second nature.

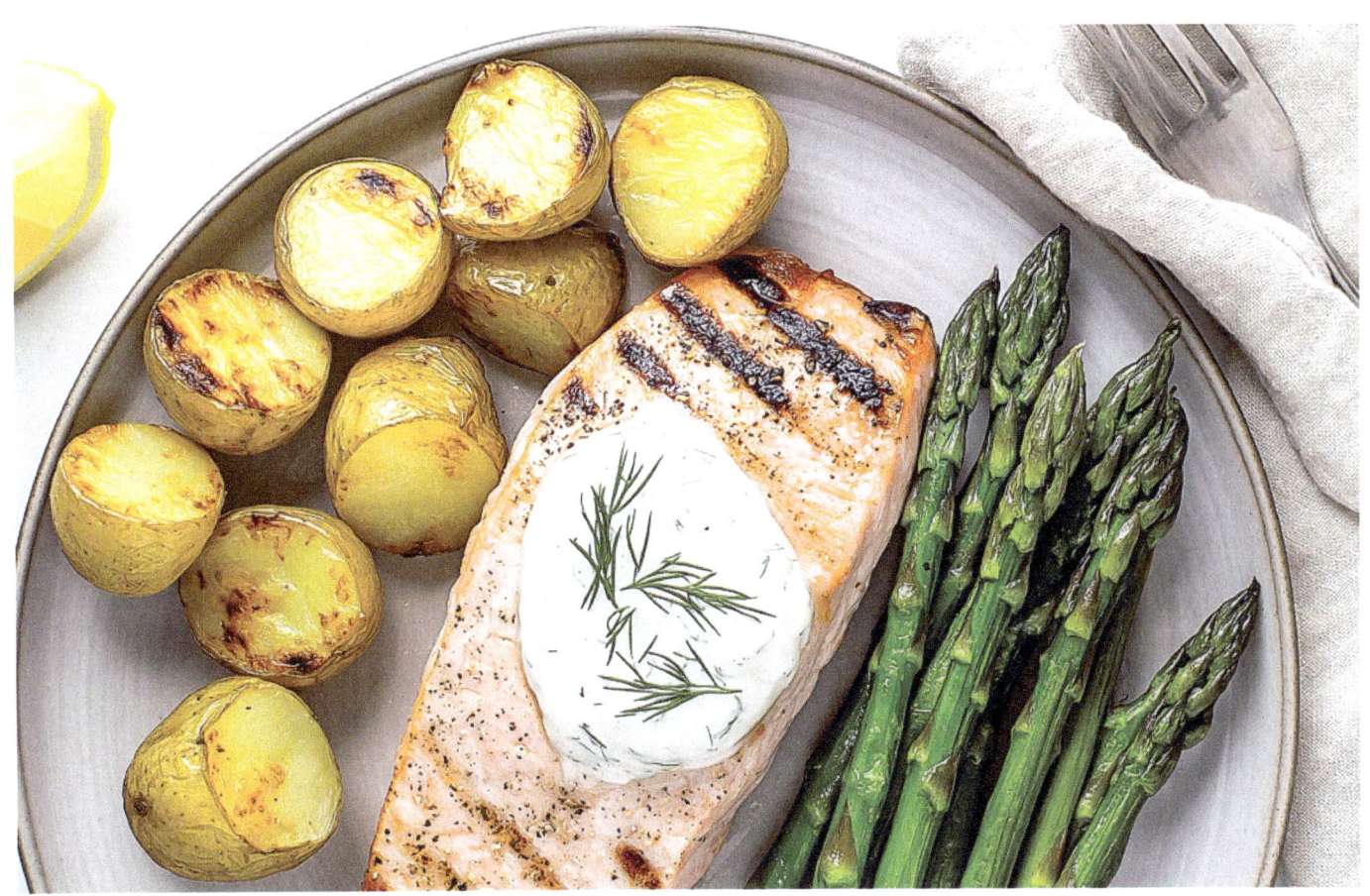

Here's an easy reference table to help you understand how much to eat in a day:

🥬	Vegetables	4-5 per day
🍌	Fruits	4-5 per day
🍞	Grains	6-8 per day
🥛	Dairy	2-3 per day
🍗	Lean protein	1-2 or per day
🧈	Fats & Oils	2-3 per day
🍦	Sweets	2-3 per week

This table shows a general recommendation for adults following the standard DASH diet (around 2,000 calories per day). Adjust portions slightly if you're more or less active, or talk to your doctor if you have specific dietary needs.

2.4 THE KEY TO BALANCE: SODIUM & SMART CHOICES

One of the reasons DASH works so well is because it doesn't ask you to eliminate foods completely—it just helps you eat smarter. By reducing a few key ingredients, you can dramatically improve your blood pressure, heart health, and overall energy.

The most important one? Sodium.

Too much salt can raise your blood pressure and make your heart work harder.

Try to stay under 2,300 mg of sodium per day—or ideally 150 mg or less per serving when preparing meals at home.

Choose low-sodium products, cook more often, and boost flavor with herbs, spices, citrus, and vinegar instead of salt.

Want to know how you're doing?

Each recipe in this book shows sodium and other key nutrients—so you'll always know what you're putting on your plate.

2.5 DASH TRAFFIC LIGHT:

I created the DASH Traffic Light to make things even easier at the grocery store or in the kitchen.

It's a simple visual guide that shows you which foods to prioritize, which to enjoy in moderation, and which to save for special occasions.

✓ **DASH Tip:**

To make it even easier, here's a quick visual guide to estimate portions—no measuring cups required:

- **Protein** = the palm of your hand
- **Grains or starches** = a cupped hand or fist
- **Fruits or veggies** = a full fist
- **Fats (like oil or butter)** = the tip of your thumb

This makes it easy to visualize your meals—whether you're at home, cooking for two, or dining out.

GREEN LIGHT CHOOSE OFTEN	YELLOW LIGHT ENJOY IN MODERATION	RED LIGHT LIMIT OR SAVE FOR SPECIAL OCCASIONS
These foods are the heart of the DASH diet. They're rich in fiber, potassium, essential nutrients and naturally low in sodium and saturated fats.	These foods can be part of a balanced DASH plate, but should be eaten in smaller portions or less frequently.	These foods are high in sodium, added sugars, or unhealthy fats. Try to limit them and keep them for special occasions.
Fresh or frozen vegetables (no salt added)	Store-bought whole wheat bread (check sodium)	Deli meats, bacon, sausages
Fresh fruits	Low-fat cheese	Ready meals or frozen dishes (with salt)
Low-sodium canned or cooked legumes	"Light" or reduced-sodium products	White bread and commercial pastries
Whole grains (like oats, brown rice, quinoa)	Whole wheat pasta	Aged or processed cheeses
White fish and oily fish	Lean cuts of chicken or pork	Salty snacks (chips, pretzels)
Unsalted nuts (in small portions)	No-salt-added sauces	Sugary sodas and drinks
Low-fat plain yogurt	Whole grain crackers or low-sodium cereals	High-sodium sauces (soy sauce, BBQ, ketchup)
Olive oil (used moderately)	Eggs or tofu (moderately)	Highly processed "diet" foods

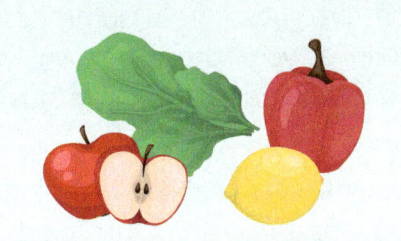

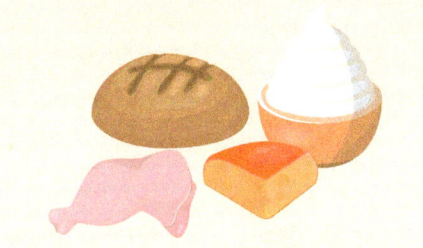

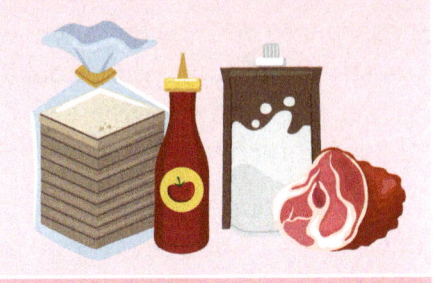

REMEMBER: No food is off-limits forever. With the DASH Traffic Light Guide, it's easier to create balance and make daily choices that support your health.

CHAPTER 3: YOUR 30-DAY DASH MEAL PLAN

3.1 HOW TO USE THE 30-DAY PLAN

This 30-Day Plan is here to help you bring the DASH lifestyle into your daily routine—flexibly and without stress. Whether you're cooking for one, two, or a small group, the meals are simple to prepare, full of flavor, and heart-friendly.

Each day includes breakfast, lunch, dinner, and an optional snack or dessert. You don't need to follow it perfectly—repeat favorites, swap meals, or skip a dish if needed. What matters most is staying consistent.

All the recipes are clearly explained in the book, so you'll never be left guessing. In some cases, you'll see "1 protein of your choice"—giving you the freedom to adapt to your tastes while staying DASH-friendly.

Missing an ingredient? No problem. You'll find helpful swaps and tips throughout the book to make adjustments easy.

Now that you're ready, let's dive into your first week of the 30-Day Plan.

DAY	BREAKFAST	LUNCH	SNACK OR DESSERT	DINNER
1	Creamy Oatmeal with Berries. Pag 22	Oven-Baked Stuffed Bell Peppers. Pag 34	Mini Carrot & Walnut Cakes. Pag 64	Lemon & Garlic Chicken with Sautéed Veggies. Pag 42
2	Tropical Mango & Coconut Smoothie Bowl. Pag 28	Zucchini Noodles with homemade DASH Pesto. Pag 36	Chocolate-Dipped Fruit Skewers. Pag 63	Warm & Rustic Beef Stew. Pag 47
3	Frittata with Spinach & Mushrooms. Pag 22	Mediterranean Chickpea Power Bowl. Pag 50	Rhubarb & Pecan Muffins. Pag 66	Hake "en Papillote" with Lemon, Zucchini & Eggplant. Pag 46
4	Greek Yogurt Parfait with Homemade Granola. Pag 23	Hearty Lentil & Veggie Soup. Pag 42	Green Revitalizing Smoothie. Pag 58	Light Tropical Chicken Curry. Pag 45
5	Avocado & Egg Breakfast Toast. Pag 28	Shakshuka with Spinach & Bell Peppers. Pag 39	DASH Tzatziki Sauce. Pag 53	Balsamic Roasted Brussels Sprouts with Walnuts. Pag 75 + 1 protein of your choice
6	Golden Toast with Ricotta & Pear Delight. Pag 29	Comforting Chicken Noodle Soup. Pag 35	Spicy DASH Trail Mix. Pag 54	Tilapia with Fresh Garden Salad & Lemon Vinaigrette. Pag 49
7	Savory Sweet Potato & Broccoli Hash. Pag 25	Whole Wheat Pasta with Roasted Veggies & Cottage Sauce. Pag 26	Light Chocolate Pudding. Pag 67	Cozy White Bean Stew with a Twist. Pag 49

DAY	BREAKFAST	LUNCH	SNACK OR DESSERT	DINNER
8	Soft-Baked Blueberry Oat Bars. Pag 25	Curried Cauliflower Steaks with Red Rice & Tzatziki. Pag 40	Sweet Potato Toasts with Cottage Cheese & Walnuts. Pag 53	Gentle Cod Curry with Veggies. Pag 48
9	Fluffy Whole Wheat Banana Pancakes. Pag 26	Hearty Lentil & Veggie Soup. Pag 30	Citrusy DASH Guacamole. Pag 56	Asian-Style Ginger Tofu & Veggie Stir-Fry. Pag 50
10	Warm Veggie Breakfast Burrito. Pag 23	Savory Turkey & Veggie Lettuce Wraps. Pag 25	American-Style Apple Crumble. Pag 67	Spiced Lentil Patties with Fresh Salad. Pag 42
11	Mini Banana Oat Loaf. Pag 24	Creamy Lemon Fettuccine with Shrimp. Pag 22	DASH-Friendly Popcorn. Pag 57	Baked Chicken with Apple & Mashed Cauliflower. Pag 47
12	Cottage Cheese Bowl with Caramelized Peach. Pag 24	Chickpea & Spinach Wraps with Creamy Yogurt Sauce. Pag 37	Chia & Mango Pudding. Pag 65	Pork Tenderloin with Fennel Sauce. Pag 48
13	Spinach & Tomato Morning Scramble. Pag 26	Zucchini Noodles with homemade DASH Pesto. Pag 36	Warm Berry Crisp with Oat Topping. Pag 68	Simple Ratatouille Bake. Pag 74 + 1 protein of your choice
14	Greek Yogurt Parfait with Homemade Granola. Pag 23	Butternut Squash Cream with Homemade Croutons. Pag 34	Cocoa & Walnut Mug Cake. Pag 66	Shrimp Stir-Fry with Colorful Veggies. Pag 36
15	Avocado & Egg Breakfast Toast. Pag 28	Zesty Grilled Chicken & Rice Salad. Pag 32	Red Antioxidant Smoothie. Pag 60	Baked Salmon with Herbed Yogurt & Greens. Pag 47
16	Frittata with Spinach & Mushrooms. Pag 22	Curried Cauliflower Steaks with Red Rice & Tzatziki. Pag 40	Warm Cinnamon-Baked Pears. Pag 62	Lemon & Garlic Chicken with Sautéed Veggies. Pag 42
17	Creamy Oatmeal with Berries. Pag 22	Stuffed Sweet Potato with Black Beans & Avocado. Pag 38	Pumpkin Pie Smoothie. Pag 60	Tender Herb-Crusted Pork with Garden Veggies. Pag 46
18	Golden Toast with Ricotta & Pear Delight. Pag 29	Whole Wheat Pasta with Roasted Veggies & Cottage Sauce. Pag 38	Homemade Baked Veggie Chips. Pag 58	Gentle Cod Curry with Veggies. Pag 48
19	Tropical Mango & Coconut Smoothie Bowl. Pag 28	Salmon & Couscous Salad with Fresh Greens. Pag 40	Creamy Hummus with Roasted Veggie Sticks. Pag 37	Eggplants with Tasty Lentils & Mushrooms. Pag 43
20	Warm Veggie Breakfast Burrito. Pag 23	Comforting Chicken Noodle Soup. Pag 35	Chocolate Pistachio Oat Cookies. Pag 65	Hake "en Papillote" with Lemon, Zucchini & Eggplant. Pag 46

DAY	BREAKFAST	LUNCH	SNACK OR DESSERT	DINNER
21	Fluffy Whole Wheat Banana Pancakes. Pag 26	Shakshuka with Spinach & Bell Peppers. Pag 39	Creamy DASH Cheesecake. Pag 64	Cozy White Bean Stew with a Twist. Pag 49
22	Soft-Baked Blueberry Oat Bars. Pag 25	Colorful Shrimp & Avocado Bowl. Pag 36	No-Bake Oat Bites with Peanut Butter & Seeds. Pag 52	Salmon with Herbed Yogurt & Roasted Veggies. Pag 45
23	Apple Cinnamon Muffins with a DASH Twist. Pag 27	Savory Turkey & Veggie Lettuce Wraps. Pag 37	Piña Colada DASH-Friendly Mocktail. Pag 59	Light Tropical Chicken Curry. Pag 45
24	Mini Carrot & Walnut Cakes. Pag 64	Creamy Lemon Fettuccine with Shrimp. Pag 39	Crunchy Seed Crackers with Herbs. Pag 56	Warm & Rustic Beef Stew. Pag 47
25	Avocado & Egg Breakfast Toast. Pag 28	Stuffed Turkey Meatballs with Spinach & Tomato. Pag 37	Tiramisu in a Cup. Pag 63	Spiced Lentil Patties with Fresh Salad. Pag 42
26	Savory Black Bean & Avocado Morning Wrap. Pag 25	Whole Wheat Pasta with Sautéed Veggies. Pag 38	Zesty Lemon Yogurt Mousse. Pag 62	Healthy Turkey & Spinach Lasagna. Pag 44
27	Greek Yogurt Parfait with Homemade Granola. Pag 23	Mediterranean Chickpea Power Bowl. Pag 50	Savory Roll-Ups with Turkey, Avocado & Spinach. Pag 57	Green Beans with Toasted Almonds & Lemon. Pag 71 + 1 protein of your choice
28	Creamy Oatmeal with Berries. Pag 22	Salmon Cakes with Sautéed Kale. Pag 35	Berry Yogurt Shake with a Twist. Pag 59	Mediterranean Chicken with Orzo & Veggies. Pag 50
29	Spinach & Tomato Morning Scramble. Pag 26	Zesty Grilled Chicken & Rice Salad. Pag 62	Mediterranean Baked Apricots with a Twist. Pag 68	Fresh Fish with Colorful Veggie Medley. Pag 43
30	Tropical Mango & Coconut Smoothie Bowl. Pag 28	Stuffed Turkey Meatballs with Spinach & Tomato. Pag 38	Chia & Mango Pudding. Pag 65	Pork Tenderloin with Fennel Sauce. Pag 48

3.3 BEFORE YOU COOK

Before diving into the recipes, here are a few things to remember. This section will help you get the most out of every meal without stress or confusion.

ABOUT RECIPE SERVINGS

This cookbook was created with your lifestyle in mind.

- Breakfasts and Snacks are designed for 2 servings, perfect for preparing something fresh without leftovers.
- Lunches, Dinners, Sides & Extras, and Desserts are designed for 4 servings—ideal for sharing with a partner, saving some for later, or hosting a guest.
- If you're cooking for one, leftovers can be stored for another day. If you're cooking for more, simply double the quantities.

It's all about making healthy eating easier, not harder.

ABOUT INGREDIENTS

We've carefully selected every ingredient to support a DASH-friendly lifestyle, while keeping things practical, affordable, and flavorful.

- You'll often find olive oil, oats, berries, leafy greens, legumes, low-fat dairy, and lean proteins.
- We've kept sodium levels low and seasoning simple.
- For more flavor, try using fresh herbs, citrus, garlic, onion, and salt-free spice blends.

FLEXIBILITY MATTERS

We know life can be unpredictable. If you're missing an ingredient—don't worry.

Each recipe includes tips to swap, adjust, or simplify depending on what you have at home.

You don't need to be a professional chef. You just need to show up for yourself with simple, nourishing choices. Every recipe you try is a step in the right direction.

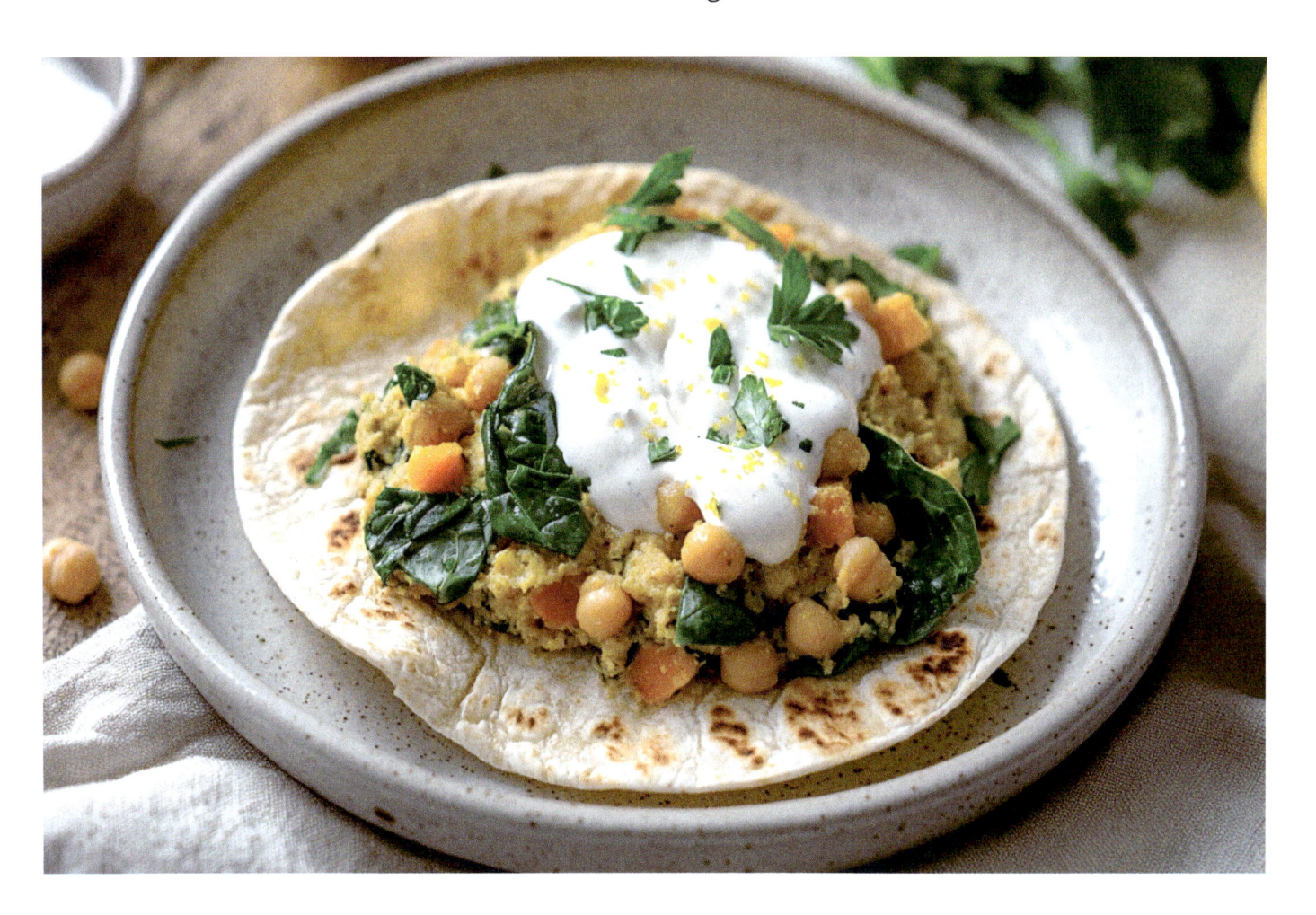

FAQS ABOUT THE 30-DAY PLAN

Before you start, it's natural to have questions.

Changing habits is a journey, and every step matters.

This section is here to answer some common doubts and help you feel more confident as you enjoy your new DASH-friendly meals.

Q: What if I miss a day or eat something less healthy?

That's completely normal! One meal won't undo your progress. Simply return to your DASH plan at the next meal and keep going. Small steps lead to lasting change.

Q: Can I swap meals or repeat my favorites?

Absolutely. Flexibility is part of the plan. Feel free to swap meals between days or repeat the ones you enjoy most. Just stay mindful of balanced portions and DASH principles.

Q: What if I'm eating out or visiting family?

Choose grilled, baked, or steamed dishes whenever possible. Ask for sauces and dressings on the side, and choose options without added salt. Focus on enjoying the company and making the best choices you can.

Q: Can I drink coffee or tea while following the DASH plan?

Yes, you can enjoy coffee and tea in moderation. Stick to 1–2 cups per day, and try to limit creamers and added sugars. And remember, staying well hydrated with plain water is just as important for your heart health.

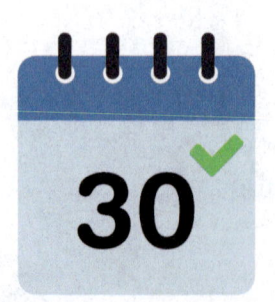

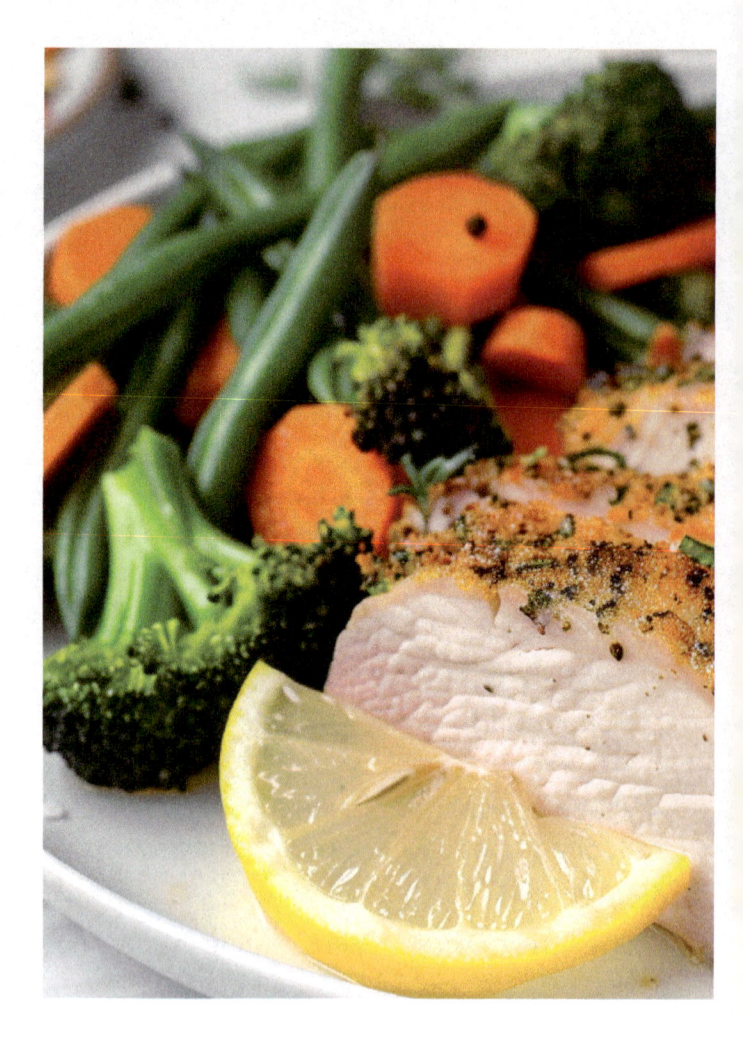

YOUR ACTION PLAN

Here's how to make the most of your 30-Day Plan:

1. **Start each day with intention.**
   Focus on nourishing your body, one meal at a time.

2. **Have a little foresight.**
   If you can, plan your meals ahead and cook a few basics (like preparing some rice or roasting vegetables) to make your week easier.

3. **Stay flexible and positive.**
   Adjust meals or swap recipes if needed—it's all part of your journey.

4. **Reflect weekly.**
   Take a few moments to notice how you're feeling, which meals you enjoyed most, and how your energy and confidence are growing.

5. **Keep moving forward.**
   Progress, not perfection, is the goal. Every small step you take supports your health and well-being.

BREAKFAST

*Start your day with heart-healthy energy and full flavor.
Simple mornings, delicious beginnings.*

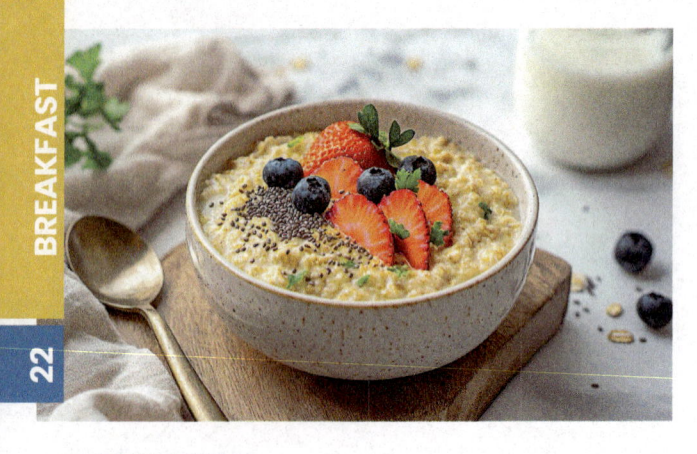

CREAMY OATMEAL WITH BERRIES

Servings: 2
Prep Time: 5 minutes
Cook Time: 5 minutes

Nutrition Facts (per serving):

Calories: 240	Carbs: 40g
Fat: 4g	Fiber: 7g
Sodium: 60mg	Protein: 9g

INGREDIENTS:
- 1 cup rolled oats (90 g)
- 2 cups skim milk or unsweetened plant-based milk (480 ml)
- ½ cup sliced strawberries (75 g)
- ½ cup blueberries (75 g)
- 1 tablespoon chia seeds (10 g)
- 1 teaspoon ground cinnamon (optional) (2 g)

INSTRUCTIONS:
1. In a medium saucepan, combine the oats and milk. Bring to medium heat.
2. Cook, stirring frequently, for about 5 minutes or until the oats are soft and creamy.
3. Divide the oatmeal into two bowls and top with strawberries, blueberries, and chia seeds.
4. Sprinkle with cinnamon if desired.

DID YOU KNOW?
Chia seeds are rich in fiber and omega-3s and you can now find them easily in most supermarkets!

FRITTATA WITH SPINACH & MUSHROOMS

Servings: 2
Prep Time: 7 minutes
Cook Time: 12 minutes

Nutrition Facts (per serving):

Calories: 165	Carbs: 2g
Fat: 11g	Fiber: 1g
Sodium: 105mg	Protein: 12g

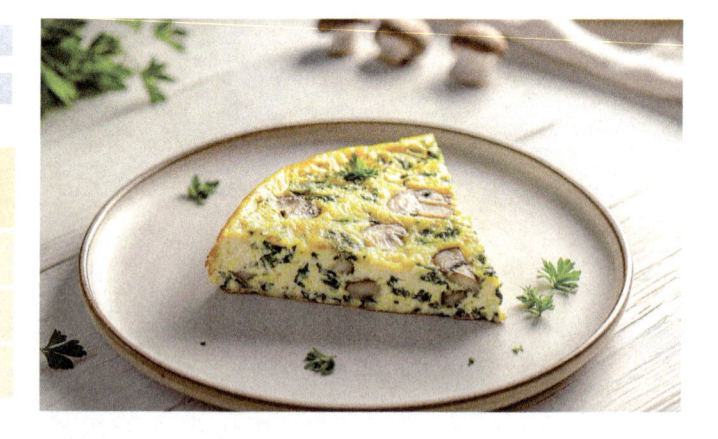

INGREDIENTS:
- 4 large eggs (200 g)
- 1 cup fresh spinach (30 g)
- 1/2 cup mushrooms (40 g)
- 1/4 cup onion (30 g)
- Olive oil spray or 1 teaspoon light olive oil (5 ml)
- 2 tablespoons low-fat milk (30 ml)
- 1 tablespoon fresh parsley (3 g)
- Black pepper to taste

INSTRUCTIONS:
1. Wash the spinach. Slice the mushrooms. Peel and chop the onion. Finely chop the parsley.
2. Lightly coat a nonstick skillet with olive oil spray and place over medium heat. Add the onion and mushrooms and sauté for 5 minutes, until soft. Add the spinach and cook for 1–2 minutes, until wilted.
3. In a bowl, whisk the eggs with the milk and black pepper. Stir in the parsley.
4. Pour the egg mixture over the vegetables in the skillet.
5. Cover the skillet with a lid or foil. Reduce heat to low and cook for 10–12 minutes or until the center is fully set.
6. Let it cool slightly, slice directly in the pan, and serve.

GREEK YOGURT PARFAIT WITH HOMEMADE GRANOLA

Servings: 2
Prep Time: 7 minutes
Cook Time: 5 minutes

Nutrition Facts (per serving):
Calories: 255 | Carbs: 24g
Fat: 10g | Fiber: 4g
Sodium: 45mg | Protein: 15g

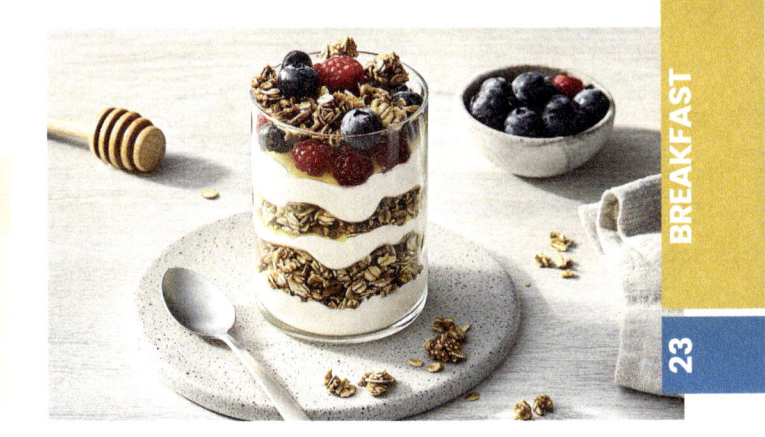

INGREDIENTS:

For the parfait:
- 1 cup plain Greek yogurt, low-fat (245 g)
- ½ cup mixed berries (75 g)
- 1 tablespoon honey (14 g)
- ½ teaspoon ground cinnamon (optional) (1 g)

For the granola:
- ½ cup rolled oats (45 g)
- 2 tablespoons nuts and seeds (20 g)
- 1 tablespoon honey (14 g)
- ½ teaspoon vanilla extract (2 ml)
- A pinch of cinnamon

INSTRUCTIONS:

1. In a dry nonstick skillet over medium heat, toast the oats and chopped nuts and seeds for 2–3 minutes, stirring constantly.
2. Add honey, vanilla extract, and a pinch of cinnamon. Stir until lightly caramelized (1–2 minutes more). Let cool.
3. In serving bowls or glasses, layer half the yogurt, then half the berries, and top with a few spoonfuls of granola.
4. Repeat the layers and finish with a drizzle of honey and cinnamon if desired.

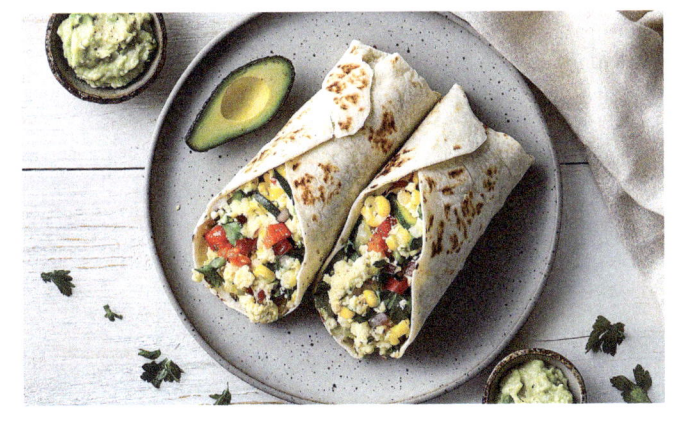

WARM VEGGIE BREAKFAST BURRITO

Servings: 2
Prep Time: 8 minutes
Cook Time: 7 minutes

Nutrition Facts (per serving):
Calories: 310 | Carbs: 22g
Fat: 17g | Fiber: 5g
Sodium: 140mg | Protein: 14g

INGREDIENTS:

- 2 small whole wheat tortillas (120 g)
- 2 large eggs
- ½ red bell pepper (60 g)
- ¼ zucchini (40 g)
- 2 tablespoons red onion (20 g)
- 2 tablespoons cooked corn (30 g)
- ¼ teaspoon ground cumin (1 g)
- 2 tablespoons shredded low-fat cheddar cheese (20 g) (optional)
- 1 tablespoon olive oil (15 ml)
- ½ avocado (optional, sliced or mashed)

INSTRUCTIONS:

1. Wash and dice the bell pepper, zucchini, and red onion.
2. In a nonstick skillet, heat the olive oil over medium heat.
3. Add the vegetables and corn, and sauté for 3–4 minutes until tender.
4. In a bowl, beat the eggs with cumin and pepper. Pour into the skillet and scramble gently until cooked.
5. Warm the tortillas briefly in the microwave or skillet.
6. Divide the egg and veggie mix between the tortillas. Add cheese if using.
7. Top with sliced or mashed avocado (optional) for a creamy, healthy finish.
8. Roll into burritos and serve.

BREAKFAST

MINI BANANA OAT LOAF

Servings: 2
Prep Time: 10 minutes
Cook Time: 20-25 minutes

Nutrition Facts (per serving):

Calories: 240	Carbs: 29g
Fat: 10g	Fiber: 5g
Sodium: 95mg	Protein: 8g

INGREDIENTS:
- 1 ripe banana (120 g)
- 1 egg
- ½ cup whole wheat flour (60 g)
- 2 tablespoons Greek yogurt, low-fat (30 g)
- 1 tablespoon olive oil (15 ml) (or unsweetened applesauce for lighter version)
- ½ teaspoon baking powder (2 g)
- ½ teaspoon ground cinnamon (1 g)
- 1 tablespoon chopped walnuts (10 g)
- ½ teaspoon vanilla extract (optional)
- 1 teaspoon seeds (e.g., poppy or chia) (optional, for topping)

INSTRUCTIONS:
1. Preheat the oven to 350°F (175°C).
2. In a bowl, mash the banana. Add the egg, yogurt, oil, and vanilla. Mix well.
3. Stir in the whole wheat flour, baking powder, and cinnamon. Fold in walnuts if using.
4. Pour the batter into two small ramekins or muffin molds. Optionally, sprinkle chopped walnuts and a few seeds on top for extra crunch and texture.
5. Bake for 20–25 minutes, or until a toothpick comes out clean.
6. Let cool slightly and serve warm.

COTTAGE CHEESE BOWL WITH CARAMELIZED PEACH

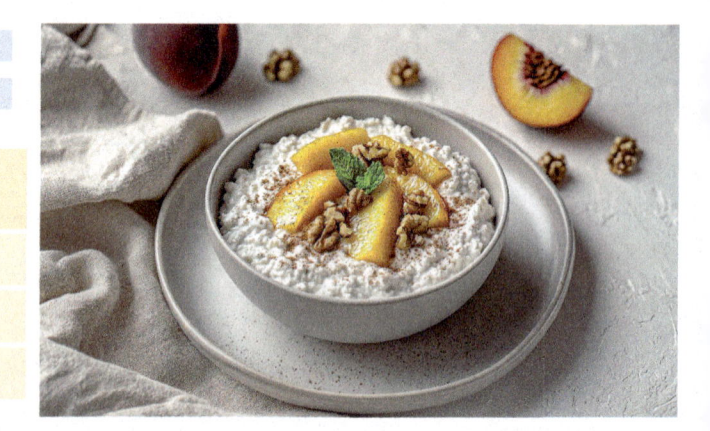

Servings: 2
Prep Time: 5 minutes
Cook Time: 6-7 minutes

Nutrition Facts (per serving):

Calories: 195	Carbs: 18g
Fat: 6g	Fiber: 2g
Sodium: 180mg	Protein: 16g

INGREDIENTS:
- 1 cup low-fat cottage cheese (225 g)
- 1 ripe peach (150 g)
- 1 teaspoon olive oil (5 ml)
- ½ teaspoon ground cinnamon (1 g)
- 1 tablespoon walnuts (10 g)
- Fresh mint to garnish

INSTRUCTIONS:
1. Slice the peach into wedges.
2. In a nonstick skillet over medium heat, add a drizzle of olive oil or use a light nonstick spray.
3. Add the peach slices and sprinkle with cinnamon. Sauté for 3–4 minutes until softened and lightly golden.
4. Divide the cottage cheese into two bowls.
5. Top with warm peaches, chopped walnuts, and fresh mint. Serve immediately.

EXPERT TIP:
Olive oil adds healthy fats, but a nonstick spray works great too if you prefer to keep it lighter.

SOFT-BAKED BLUEBERRY OAT BARS

Servings: 2
Prep Time: 10 minutes
Cook Time: 20-25 minutes

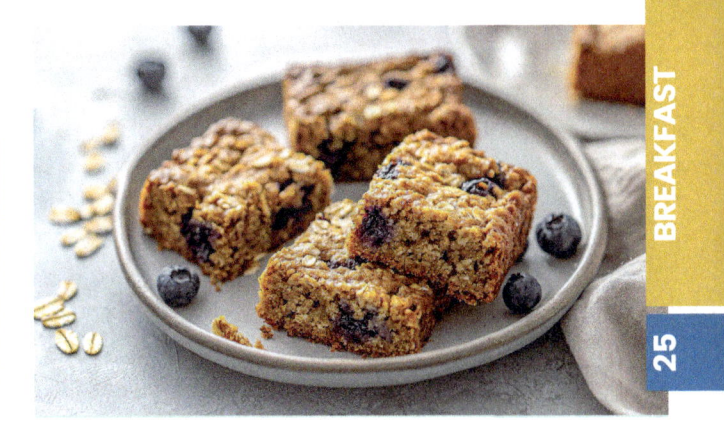

Nutrition Facts (per serving):
- Calories: 240
- Fat: 8g
- Sodium: 90mg
- Carbs: 32g
- Fiber: 5g
- Protein: 6g

INGREDIENTS:
- 1 ripe banana (120 g)
- 1 tablespoon olive oil or canola oil (15 ml)
- ½ cup rolled oats (45 g)
- ¼ cup whole wheat flour (30 g)
- 1 egg
- ½ teaspoon baking powder (2 g)
- ½ teaspoon ground cinnamon (1 g)
- ½ teaspoon vanilla extract (optional)
- ½ cup fresh or frozen blueberries (70 g)

INSTRUCTIONS:
1. Preheat oven to 350°F (175°C).
2. In a bowl, mash the banana. Add egg, oil, and vanilla. Mix well.
3. Add oats, flour, baking powder, and cinnamon. Stir until fully combined.
4. Gently fold in the blueberries.
5. Pour mixture into a small lined or greased baking dish (approx. 6x6 in / 15x15 cm).
6. Bake for 20-25 minutes or until set and lightly golden.
7. Let cool, then slice into 4 bars. Serve or store.

EXPERT TIP:
Soft, fruity, and full of fiber—these bars are great for a quick snack or light breakfast.

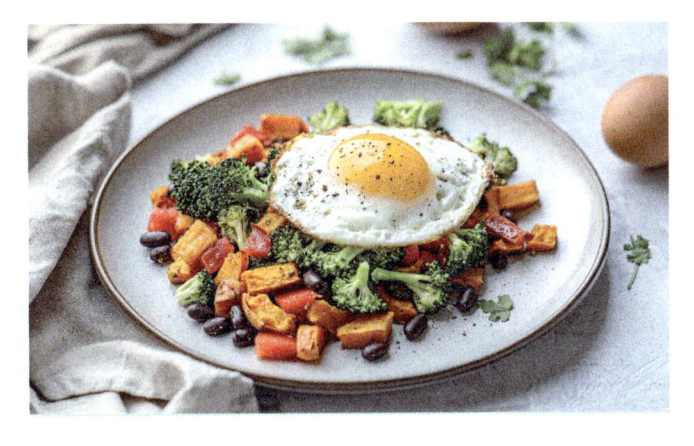

SAVORY SWEET POTATO & BROCCOLI HASH

Servings: 2
Prep Time: 10 minutes
Cook Time: 15 minutes

Nutrition Facts (per serving):
- Calories: 240
- Fat: 4g
- Sodium: 60mg
- Carbs: 40g
- Fiber: 7g
- Protein: 9g

INGREDIENTS:
- 1 medium sweet potato (200 g)
- 1 cup broccoli florets (100 g)
- 1 small red bell pepper (60 g)
- 1/2 cup black beans, cooked (120 g)
- 2 large eggs
- 1 tablespoon olive oil (15 ml) (or nonstick spray)
- ¼ teaspoon smoked paprika (1 g)
- Salt and pepper to taste

INSTRUCTIONS:
1. Peel and dice the sweet potato. Boil in a small pot of water for 6-7 minutes, until slightly tender. Drain and set aside.
2. In a nonstick skillet, add olive oil or spray and heat over medium.
3. Add the bell pepper and sweet potato. Sauté for 5-6 minutes, stirring occasionally.
4. Add the black beans and broccoli. Cook for 3-4 minutes, until the broccoli is tender and everything is heated through. Season with paprika, salt, and pepper.
5. In a separate pan, cook the eggs to your liking (fried, scrambled, etc.).
6. Serve the hash onto plates and top each portion with a cooked egg.

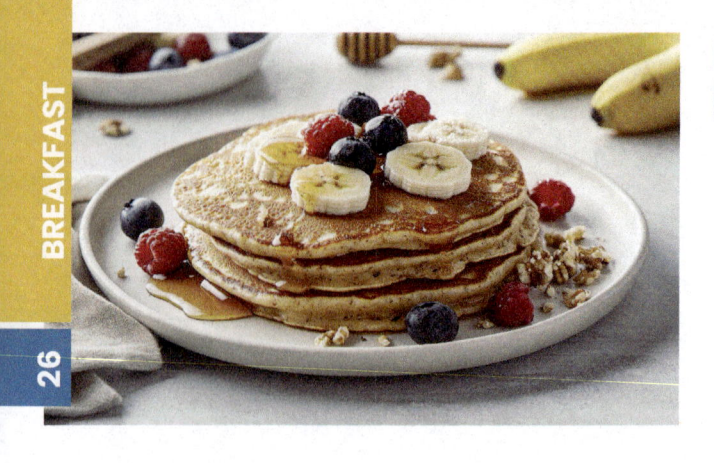

FLUFFY WHOLE WHEAT BANANA PANCAKES

Servings: 2
Prep Time: 10 minutes
Cook Time: 10 minutes

Nutrition Facts (per serving):

Calories: 260	Carbs: 36g
Fat: 8g	Fiber: 5g
Sodium: 95mg	Protein: 9g

INGREDIENTS:
- 1 ripe banana (120 g)
- 1 egg
- ½ cup whole wheat flour (60 g)
- ½ teaspoon baking powder (2 g)
- ½ teaspoon ground cinnamon (1 g)
- ⅓ cup low-fat milk (80 ml)
- 1 teaspoon olive oil (5 ml)
- Optional toppings: sliced banana, fresh berries or other fruits, unsalted chopped nuts or a drizzle of honey

INSTRUCTIONS:
1. In a bowl, mash the banana. Add the egg and whisk until combined.
2. Add the flour, baking powder, cinnamon, and milk. Stir to form a smooth batter.
3. Heat a nonstick skillet over medium heat and lightly brush with olive oil.
4. Pour small amounts of batter to form 4 pancakes. Cook for 2–3 minutes per side until golden brown.
5. Serve warm with optional toppings.

STORAGE TIP:
Freeze any leftover pancakes in an airtight bag. Toast them for a quick and heart-healthy breakfast anytime.

SPINACH & TOMATO MORNING SCRAMBLE

Servings: 2
Prep Time: 5 minutes
Cook Time: 5 minutes

Nutrition Facts (per serving):

Calories: 190	Carbs: 4 g
Fat: 12 g	Fiber: 1 g
Sodium: 140 mg	Protein: 15 g

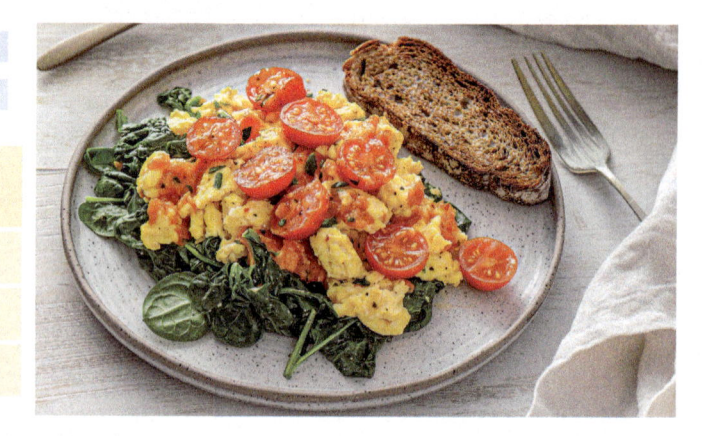

INGREDIENTS:
- 4 large eggs
- 1 cup fresh spinach (30 g)
- 6–8 cherry tomatoes (120 g)
- 2 tablespoons low-fat milk (30 ml) (optional)
- 1 teaspoon olive oil (5 ml)
- Black pepper, to taste

INSTRUCTIONS:
1. Crack the eggs into a bowl and beat with a fork. Add milk and black pepper.
2. Wash and halve the cherry tomatoes. Rinse and roughly chop the spinach.
3. In a nonstick skillet over medium heat, warm the olive oil.
4. Add the cherry tomatoes and cook for 2 minutes until slightly softened.
5. Add the spinach and stir until just wilted.
6. Pour in the eggs and gently scramble until fully cooked. Serve warm.

APPLE CINNAMON MUFFINS WITH A DASH TWIST

Servings: 2

Prep Time: 10 minutes

Cook Time: 18–20 minutes

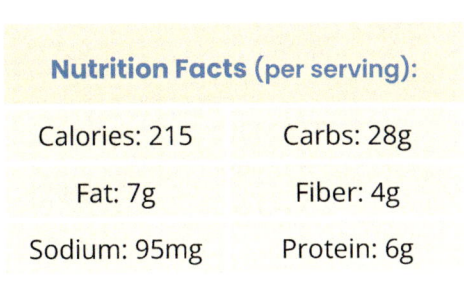

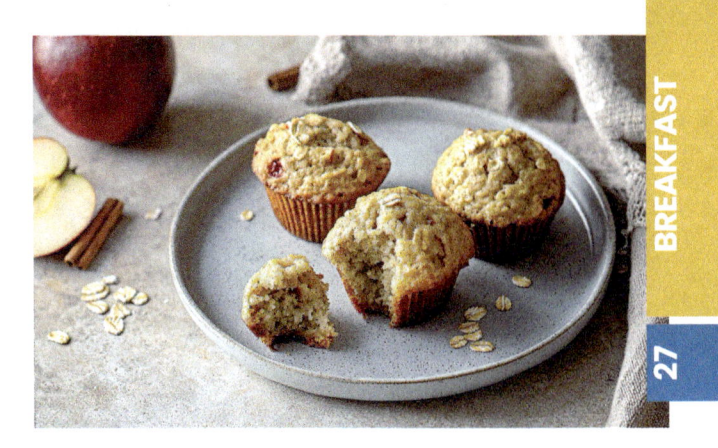

Nutrition Facts (per serving):
- Calories: 215
- Carbs: 28g
- Fat: 7g
- Fiber: 4g
- Sodium: 95mg
- Protein: 6g

INGREDIENTS:
- ½ cup rolled oats (45 g)
- ¼ cup whole wheat flour (30 g)
- 1 small apple (120 g)
- 1 egg
- 2 tablespoons unsweetened applesauce (30 g)
- 2 tablespoons low-fat milk (30 ml)
- ½ teaspoon baking powder (2 g)
- ½ teaspoon ground cinnamon (1 g)
- ½ teaspoon vanilla extract (optional)
- 1 tablespoon chopped walnuts (10 g) (optional)

INSTRUCTIONS:
1. Preheat the oven to 350°F (175°C).
2. In a bowl, whisk together the egg, milk, applesauce, and vanilla.
3. Add oats, flour, baking powder, and cinnamon. Stir until combined.
4. Fold in the peeled and diced apple and walnuts, if using.
5. Spoon the batter into 4 mini muffin molds or silicone cups. Optionally, sprinkle a few rolled oats on top for a rustic finish.
6. Bake for 18–20 minutes, or until golden and a toothpick comes out clean.
7. Let cool slightly before serving.

PUMPKIN HAZELNUT BREAKFAST LOAF

Makes: 1 small loaf (6 slices)

Prep Time: 10 minutes

Cook Time: 40 minutes

Nutrition Facts (per serving):
- Calories: 200
- Carbs: 24g
- Fat: 9g
- Fiber: 3g
- Sodium: 125mg
- Protein: 5g

INGREDIENTS:
- 1 cup unsalted canned pumpkin
- 2 large eggs
- 1/4 cup olive oil (60 ml)
- 1/3 cup low-fat milk (80 ml)
- 1/3 cup hazelnuts (40 g)
- 3/4 cup whole wheat flour (90 g)
- 1/2 cup oat flour (60 g)
- 1 teaspoon baking powder (4 g)
- 1/2 teaspoon baking soda (2 g)
- 1 teaspoon ground cinnamon (2 g)
- 1/4 cup maple syrup (60 ml)

INSTRUCTIONS:
1. Preheat the oven to 180°C (350°F). Line a small loaf pan with parchment paper.
2. In a large bowl, whisk the eggs, pumpkin, olive oil, milk, and maple syrup until smooth.
3. In another bowl, combine the flours, baking powder, baking soda, and cinnamon.
4. Add the dry ingredients to the wet mixture and stir until just combined. Fold in the chopped hazelnuts.
5. Pour the batter into the prepared pan, spread evenly, and sprinkle extra chopped hazelnuts on top for a delicious crunchy finish.
6. Bake for 35–40 minutes, or until a toothpick inserted in the center comes out clean. Let cool before slicing and serving.

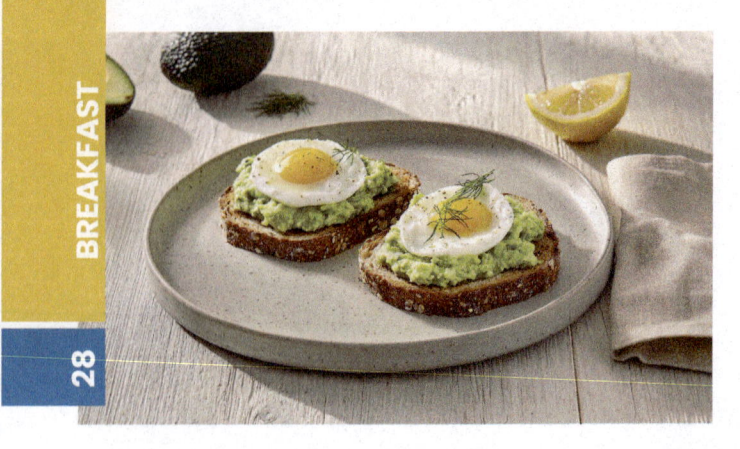

AVOCADO & EGG BREAKFAST TOAST WITH LEMON & DILL

Servings: 2
Prep Time: 5 minutes
Cook Time: 5 minutes

Nutrition Facts (per serving):

Calories: 240	Fiber: 6 g
Protein: 12 g	Fat: 14 g
Carbs: 18 g	Sodium: 160 mg

INGREDIENTS:
- 2 slices whole grain bread (60 g)
- ½ ripe avocado (75 g)
- 2 large eggs
- ½ teaspoon fresh lemon juice (2 ml)
- Fresh dill (3 g)
- Black pepper, to taste
- Olive oil cooking spray
- A few fresh dill leaves

INSTRUCTIONS:
1. Toast the bread slices until lightly golden and crispy.
2. In a bowl, mash the avocado gently with lemon juice and freshly chopped dill. Set aside.
3. Cook the eggs to your liking, poached or lightly fried with minimal oil.
4. Spread the avocado mixture evenly on each slice of toast.
5. Top each avocado toast with a cooked egg, and season lightly with black pepper and dill.
6. Serve immediately and enjoy warm.

EXPERT TIP:
Lemon juice boosts flavor and keeps the avocado from browning—perfect for a fresh, vibrant breakfast.

TROPICAL MANGO & COCONUT SMOOTHIE BOWL

Servings: 2
Prep Time: 7 minutes
Cook Time: -

Nutrition Facts (per serving):

Calories: 230	Fiber: 4 g
Protein: 6 g	Fat: 9 g
Carbs: 30 g	Sodium: 45 mg

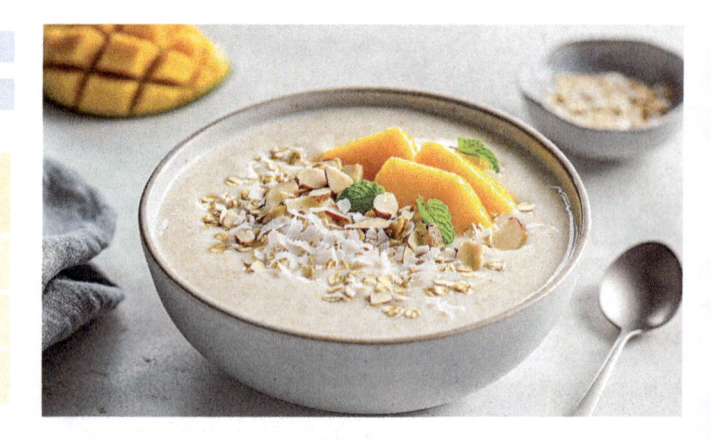

INGREDIENTS:
- 1 small ripe banana (120 g)
- 1 cup frozen mango chunks (160 g)
- ½ cup plain low-fat yogurt (120 g)
- ¼ cup light coconut milk (60 ml)
- 2 tablespoons rolled oats (20 g)
- 1 tablespoon chopped almonds (10 g)
- 1 tablespoon shredded unsweetened coconut (7 g)
- A few thin mango slices and mint leaves for topping (optional)

INSTRUCTIONS:
1. Add banana, frozen mango, yogurt, coconut milk, and oats to a blender.
2. Blend until smooth and creamy.
3. Pour into two bowls and smooth the top.
4. Sprinkle with chopped almonds and shredded coconut.
5. Add extra mango slices and mint leaves for garnish, if desired.
6. Serve immediately and enjoy chilled.

SAVORY BLACK BEAN & AVOCADO MORNING WRAP

Servings: 2
Prep Time: 10 minutes
Cook Time: 5 minutes

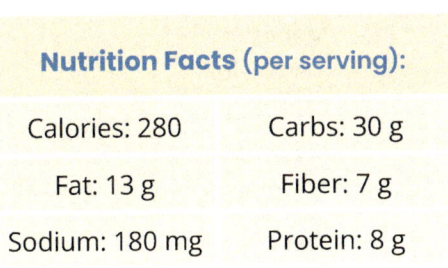

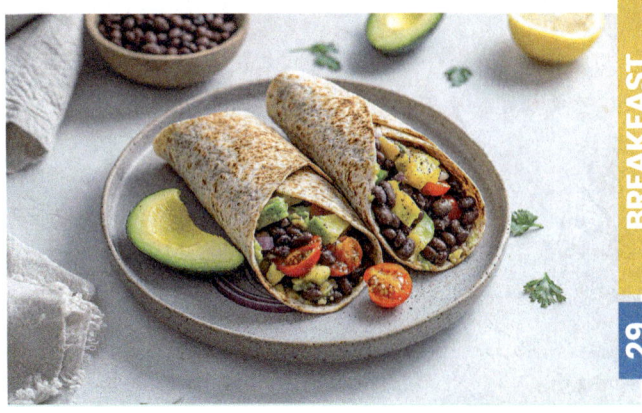

Nutrition Facts (per serving):
- Calories: 280
- Fat: 13 g
- Sodium: 180 mg
- Carbs: 30 g
- Fiber: 7 g
- Protein: 8 g

INGREDIENTS:
- 2 small whole wheat tortillas (120 g)
- ½ cup cooked black beans (85 g)
- ¼ avocado (35 g)
- ½ cup cherry tomatoes (75 g)
- ½ red onion (about 30 g)
- 1 small yellow bell pepper (about 30 g)
- 1 tablespoon olive oil (15 ml) or olive oil spray
- 1 tablespoon lemon juice (15 ml)
- Black pepper to taste

INSTRUCTIONS:
1. Halve the cherry tomatoes, finely slice the red onion, and dice the yellow bell pepper.
2. In a pan, heat a bit of oil and sauté the onion, tomatoes, and yellow bell pepper for 3–4 minutes until softened.
3. Add the black beans to the pan and stir for another 1–2 minutes to warm.
4. Remove from heat and toss with lemon juice and black pepper.
5. Warm the tortillas and fill each with the bean and veggie mixture, plus the diced avocado.
6. Wrap tightly and serve immediately.

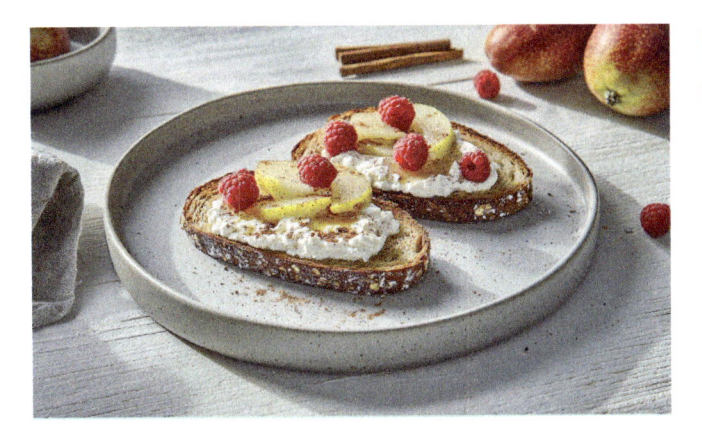

GOLDEN TOAST WITH RICOTTA & PEAR DELIGHT

Servings: 2
Prep Time: 7 minutes
Cook Time: 5 minutes

Nutrition Facts (per serving):
- Calories: 240
- Fat: 8 g
- Sodium: 110 mg
- Carbs: 30 g
- Fiber: 4 g
- Protein: 10 g

INGREDIENTS:
- 2 slices whole wheat bread (60 g)
- ½ cup low-fat ricotta cheese (120 g)
- 1 ripe pear (150 g)
- 6–8 fresh raspberries or blackberries (30 g)
- 2 teaspoons walnuts or pecans (optional, 10 g)
- ¼ teaspoon cinnamon (1 g)
- 1 teaspoon maple syrup (optional, 5 ml)
- Olive oil spray

INSTRUCTIONS:
1. Lightly spray a skillet with olive oil and heat over medium. Sauté the pear slices for 3–4 minutes until lightly golden and softened.
2. Toast the bread slices until crisp.
3. Spread ricotta over each toast, then layer with the warm pear slices.
4. Top with berries, chopped nuts (if using), and a sprinkle of cinnamon.
5. Drizzle a bit of maple syrup if desired, and serve warm.

DASH TIP:
Toasting pear enhances its sweetness naturally. Combine with grains and protein for a balanced, energizing breakfast.

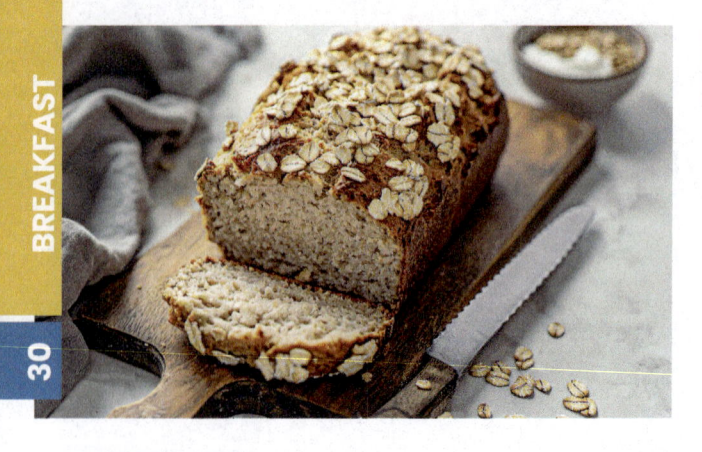

HEARTY SEEDED WHOLE GRAIN BREAD

Makes: 1 small loaf (8 slices)
Prep Time: 10 minutes
Cook Time: 35 minutes

Nutrition Facts (per serving):

Calories: 180	Carbs: 22g
Fat: 7g	Fiber: 4g
Sodium: 170mg	Protein: 7g

INGREDIENTS:

- 1 ½ cups whole wheat flour (180 g)
- ½ cup rolled oats (50 g)
- 2 teaspoons baking powder (8 g)
- ½ teaspoon baking soda (2 g)
- 1 cup plain low-fat yogurt (240 g)
- 1 egg
- 2 tablespoons olive oil (30 ml)
- 2 tablespoons mixed seeds (e.g., flax-seeds, sunflower seeds) (20 g)

INSTRUCTIONS:

1. Preheat the oven to 350°F (175°C) and line a small loaf pan with parchment paper.
2. In a large bowl, mix the flour, oats, baking powder, baking soda, and seeds.
3. In another bowl, whisk the yogurt, egg, and olive oil until smooth.
4. Combine the wet and dry ingredients, stirring gently until just incorporated.
5. Pour the batter into the prepared pan, smooth the top, and sprinkle with rolled oats.
6. Bake for 35 minutes, or until golden and a toothpick inserted comes out clean. Cool before slicing.

EASY OLIVE & HERB BREAD

Makes: 1 small loaf (8 slices)
Prep Time: 10 minutes
Cook Time: 35 minutes

Nutrition Facts (per serving):

Calories: 185	Carbs: 20g
Fat: 8g	Fiber: 3g
Sodium: 140mg	Protein: 6g

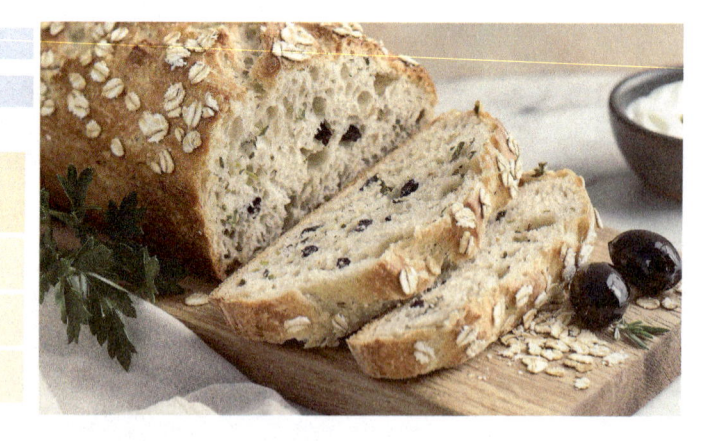

INGREDIENTS:

- Ingredients
- 1 ½ cups whole wheat flour (180 g)
- 2 teaspoons baking powder (8 g)
- ½ teaspoon dried oregano
- ¼ teaspoon garlic powder
- 1 cup plain low-fat yogurt (240 g)
- 1 egg
- 2 tablespoons olive oil (30 ml)
- ¼ cup chopped black olives, rinsed (35 g)
- Black pepper to taste
- Optional: 1 tablespoon chopped parsley

INSTRUCTIONS:

1. Preheat oven to 350°F (175°C). Grease a small loaf pan or line with parchment paper.
2. In a large bowl, mix flour, baking powder, oregano, garlic powder, and pepper.
3. In another bowl, whisk yogurt, egg, and olive oil.
4. Stir wet and dry ingredients together until combined, then fold in olives and parsley.
5. Pour the batter into the pan and smooth the top.
6. Bake for 35–40 minutes until firm and golden. Let cool before slicing.

LUNCH

*Midday meals that nourish, satisfy, and keep you going strong.
Light, balanced, and full of life—perfect for your active day.*

LUNCH

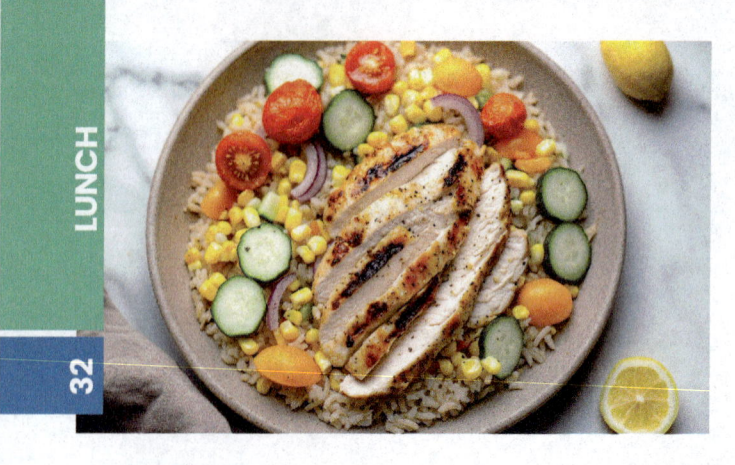

32

ZESTY GRILLED CHICKEN & RICE SALAD

Servings: 4
Prep Time: 15 minutes
Cook Time: 25 minutes

Nutrition Facts (per serving):

Calories: 320	Carbs: 20g
Fat: 9g	Fiber: 5g
Sodium: 150mg	Protein: 28g

INGREDIENTS:

- 300 g grilled chicken breast
- 1 cup cooked brown rice (200 g)
- 1 cup corn (120 g)
- 1 cup cherry tomatoes (150 g)
- 1/2 cup cucumber (75 g)
- 1/4 cup red onion (30 g)
- 1 tablespoon olive oil (15 ml)
- 1 tablespoon lemon juice (5 ml)
- 1 teaspoon dried oregano (1 g)
- Black pepper to taste

INSTRUCTIONS:

1. Grill the chicken breast and slice it thinly.
2. Cook the brown rice according to package instructions, then set aside to cool.
3. Cut the cherry tomatoes in half, dice the cucumber, and finely chop the red onion.
4. In a large bowl, combine the rice, grilled chicken, corn, cherry tomatoes, cucumber, and red onion.
5. Drizzle with olive oil and lemon juice, then sprinkle with oregano and black pepper. Toss to combine.
6. Serve chilled or at room temperature.

MEDITERRANEAN CHICKPEA POWER BOWL

Servings: 4
Prep Time: 10 minutes
Cook Time: 10 minutes

Nutrition Facts (per serving):

Calories: 360	Carbs: 40g
Fat: 13g	Fiber: 7g
Sodium: 140mg (mostly from cheese, optional)	Protein: 12g

INGREDIENTS:

- 1 can (15 oz / 425 g) low-sodium chickpeas
- 1 cup cooked whole grains (such as brown rice, quinoa, or bulgur) (200 g)
- 1 cup cucumber (130 g)
- 1 cup cherry tomatoes (150 g)
- ½ red onion (60 g)
- ½ cup light fresh cheese (60 g) (optional)
- 2 tablespoons olive oil (30 ml)
- Juice of 1 lemon
- 1 teaspoon dried oregano
- Pepper to taste (optional)

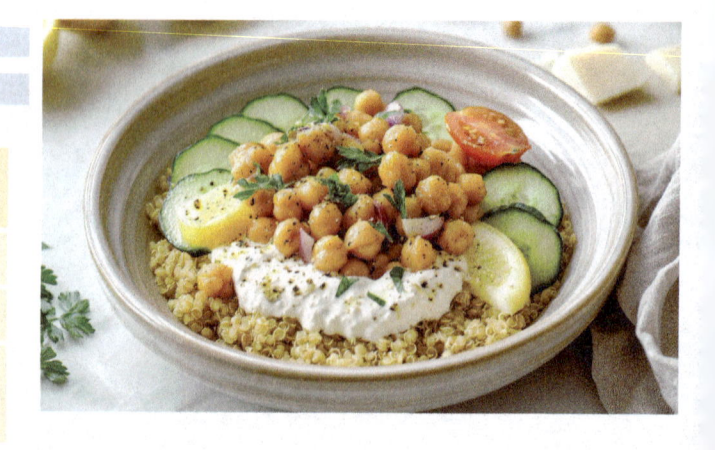

INSTRUCTIONS:

1. Slice the cucumber and cherry tomatoes. Thinly slice the red onion.
2. In a skillet, warm the chickpeas over medium heat with olive oil, lemon juice, oregano, and a pinch of pepper for 5–6 minutes, just until fragrant.
3. Cut or crumble the fresh cheese if using.
4. In a large bowl, combine the cooked grains, warm chickpeas, vegetables, and cheese.
5. Drizzle with a little extra lemon juice before serving.

HEARTY LENTIL & VEGETABLE STEW

Servings: 4
Prep Time: 10 minutes
Cook Time: 30 minutes

Nutrition Facts (per serving):
- Calories: 290
- Carbs: 38g
- Fat: 6g
- Fiber: 11g
- Sodium: 180mg
- Protein: 16g

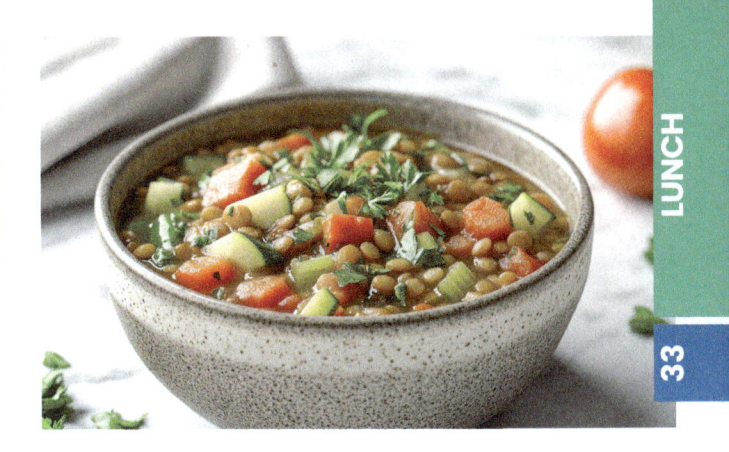

INGREDIENTS:
- 1 tablespoon olive oil (15 ml)
- 1 small onion (70 g)
- 2 garlic cloves (6 g)
- 2 carrots (120 g)
- 2 celery stalks (100 g)
- 1 zucchini (120 g)
- 1 cup dried brown or green lentils, rinsed (200 g)
- 2 medium fresh tomatoes (300 g)
- 4 cups low-sodium vegetable broth (950 ml)
- 1 teaspoon dried oregano
- 1 teaspoon dried thyme
- Pepper to taste (optional)

INSTRUCTIONS:
1. Cut the onion, carrots, celery, zucchini, and tomatoes into small pieces. Finely mince the garlic.
2. In a large pot, heat the olive oil over medium heat. Add the onion, garlic, carrots, and celery. Cook for 5–6 minutes, until slightly softened.
3. Stir in the zucchini, tomatoes, lentils, broth, oregano, thyme and pepper.
4. Bring to a boil, then reduce heat to low. Cover and simmer for 25–30 minutes, or until lentils are tender.
5. Remove the bay leaf before serving. If desired, stir in the lemon juice for a fresh finishing touch.

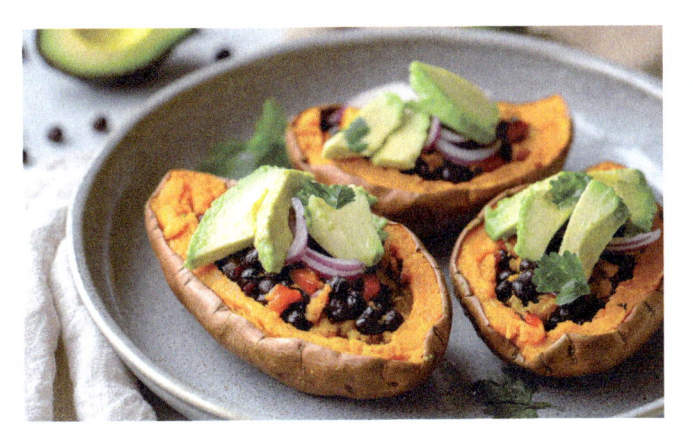

STUFFED SWEET POTATO WITH BLACK BEANS & AVOCADO

Servings: 4
Prep Time: 10 minutes
Cook Time: 30 minutes

Nutrition Facts (per serving):
- Calories: 235
- Carbs: 39g
- Fat: 4g
- Fiber: 7g
- Sodium: 60mg
- Protein: 9g

INGREDIENTS:
- 4 medium sweet potatoes (900 g)
- 1 tablespoon olive oil (15 ml)
- 1 small red onion (70 g)
- 1 can (15 oz / 425 g) no-salt-added black beans
- 1 medium red bell pepper (120 g)
- 1 teaspoon ground cumin
- ½ teaspoon smoked paprika
- Juice of 1 lime (30 ml)
- 1 avocado (150 g)

INSTRUCTIONS:
1. Preheat oven to 400°F (200°C). Wash sweet potatoes, pierce with a fork, and bake for 30–35 minutes, until soft.
2. Meanwhile, dice onion and bell pepper. Rinse black beans to remove excess sodium.
3. Heat olive oil in a skillet over medium heat. Sauté onion and pepper for 5 minutes.
4. Add beans, cumin, paprika, and a splash of water. Cook 4 more minutes. Finish with lime juice.
5. Slice sweet potatoes open and mash the center. Fill with bean mix, top with avocado, and serve.

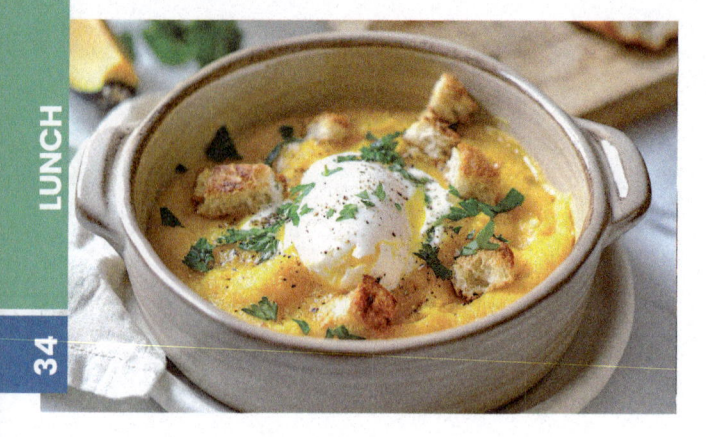

BUTTERNUT SQUASH CREAM WITH HOMEMADE CROUTONS

Servings: 4
Prep Time: 10 minutes
Cook Time: 25 minutes

Nutrition Facts (per serving):

Calories: 290	Fiber: 6 g
Protein: 10 g	Total Fat: 10 g
Carbs: 35 g	Sodium: 220 mg

INGREDIENTS:
- 1 medium butternut squash (about 2 lb / 900 g)
- 1 medium onion (200 g)
- 2 small potatoes (260 g)
- 4 cups low-sodium vegetable broth (960 ml)
- 1 tablespoon olive oil (15 ml)
- 4 eggs
- 4 slices whole grain bread
- 1 pinch ground nutmeg (optional)
- Fresh parsley to garnish (optional)
- 1 teaspoon vinegar (for poaching eggs)

INSTRUCTIONS:
1. Peel and dice the squash, onion, and potatoes.
2. In a large pot, heat the olive oil over medium heat and sauté the onion for 3–4 minutes until soft.
3. Add squash and potatoes, pour in the broth, bring to a boil, then simmer for 20 minutes.
4. Toast the bread cubes in a dry skillet until golden and crispy.
5. Poach the eggs: boil water, add a splash of vinegar, create a whirlpool and cook each egg for 3 minutes.
6. Blend the soup until smooth then add nutmeg if desired, and serve topped with a poached egg, croutons, and parsley.

OVEN-BAKED STUFFED BELL PEPPERS

Servings: 4
Prep Time: 15 minutes
Cook Time: 35 minutes

Nutrition Facts (per serving):

Calories: 240	Carbs: 32g
Fat: 8g	Fiber: 6g
Sodium: 150mg	Protein: 7g

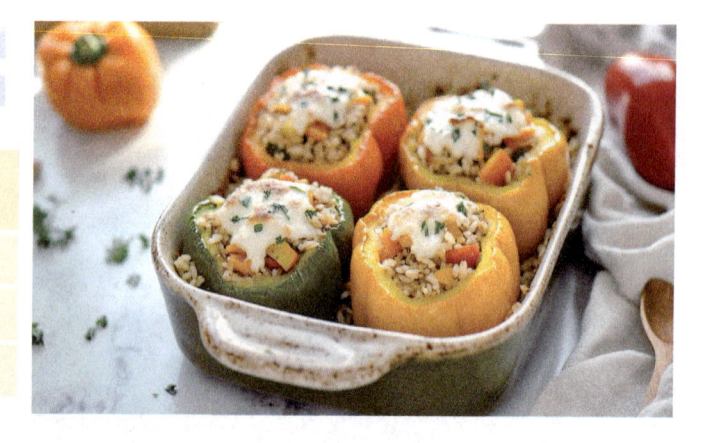

INGREDIENTS:
- 4 large bell peppers (any color)
- 1 tablespoon olive oil (15 ml)
- 1 small onion (70 g)
- 1 medium zucchini (120 g)
- 1 garlic clove (3 g)
- 1 cup cooked brown rice or quinoa (180 g)
- 1 can (15 oz / 425 g) no-salt-added diced tomatoes
- 1 teaspoon dried oregano
- ½ teaspoon ground cumin
- Pepper to taste (optional)
- 2 tablespoons light mozzarella (optional)

INSTRUCTIONS:
1. Preheat the oven to 375°F (190°C). Cut the tops off the peppers, remove seeds, and place upright in a baking dish. Pre-bake for 10 minutes.
2. Dice the onion and zucchini. Mince the garlic. Sauté everything in olive oil for 5–6 minutes.
3. In a bowl, mix the sautéed veggies with cooked rice or quinoa, tomatoes, oregano, cumin, and pepper.
4. Fill the pre-baked peppers with the mixture. Top with cheese if using.
5. Cover with foil and bake for 20 minutes. Uncover and bake 5 more minutes to lightly brown the tops.

COMFORTING CHICKEN NOODLE SOUP

Servings: 4
Prep Time: 10 minutes
Cook Time: 25 minutes

Nutrition Facts (per serving):
- Calories: 260
- Fat: 7g
- Sodium: 190mg
- Carbs: 25g
- Fiber: 4g
- Protein: 22g

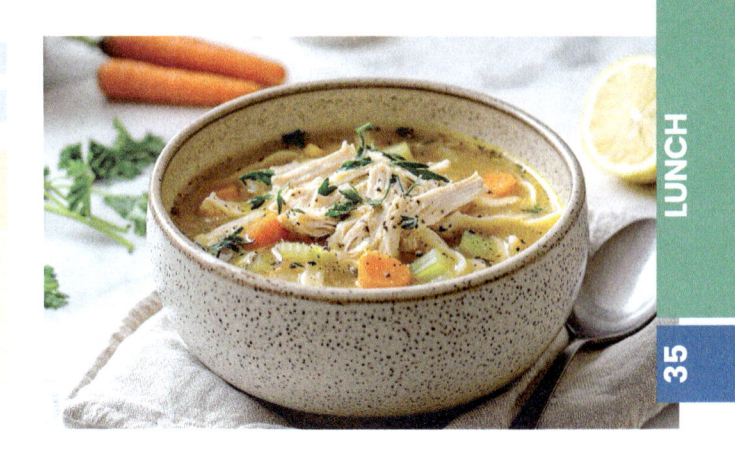

INGREDIENTS:
- 1 tablespoon olive oil (15 ml)
- 1 small onion (70 g)
- 2 medium carrots (120 g)
- 2 celery stalks (100 g)
- 1 garlic clove (3 g)
- 6 cups low-sodium chicken broth (1.4 L)
- 1 cup cooked chicken breast (140 g)
- 1 cup whole grain noodles or whole wheat pasta (85 g, dry weight)
- 1 teaspoon dried thyme
- ½ teaspoon dried parsley
- Pepper to taste (optional)

INSTRUCTIONS:
1. Dice the onion, carrots, and celery. Mince the garlic.
2. In a large pot, heat olive oil over medium heat. Sauté the onion, carrots, celery, and garlic for 5–6 minutes until softened.
3. Add the chicken broth, thyme, parsley, and pepper. Bring to a gentle boil.
4. Add the noodles and cook according to package instructions, until tender.
5. Stir in the shredded chicken and simmer for 3–4 more minutes until heated through.
6. Remove from heat and add a splash of lemon juice if desired. Serve warm.

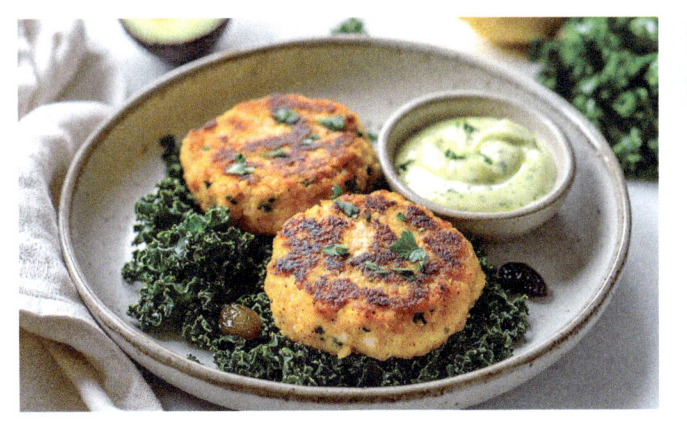

SALMON CAKES WITH SAUTÉED KALE

Servings: 4
Prep Time: 15 minutes
Cook Time: 10 minutes

Nutrition Facts (per serving):
- Calories: 285
- Protein: 25 g
- Carbs: 10 g
- Fiber: 3 g
- Total Fat: 16 g
- Sodium: 180 mg

INGREDIENTS:
- 2 cans no-salt-added salmon (approx. 300 g total)
- 1 large egg
- ⅓ cup whole wheat breadcrumbs (40 g)
- 2 tablespoons plain low-fat yogurt (30 g)
- 2 tablespoons red or yellow onion (20 g)
- Black pepper to taste
- 1 teaspoon olive oil (5 ml)
- 2 cups kale (60 g)
- 1 tablespoon raisins (10 g)

INSTRUCTIONS:
1. In a bowl, mix the salmon, egg, breadcrumbs, yogurt, onion, and pepper until combined.
2. Chill the mixture for 10 minutes.
3. Heat ½ teaspoon olive oil in a skillet. Shape 8 patties and cook for 3–4 minutes per side, until golden. Set aside.
4. In the same skillet, sauté kale and raisins with the remaining oil for 3–4 minutes, until wilted.
5. Serve 2 patties per person with warm sautéed kale.

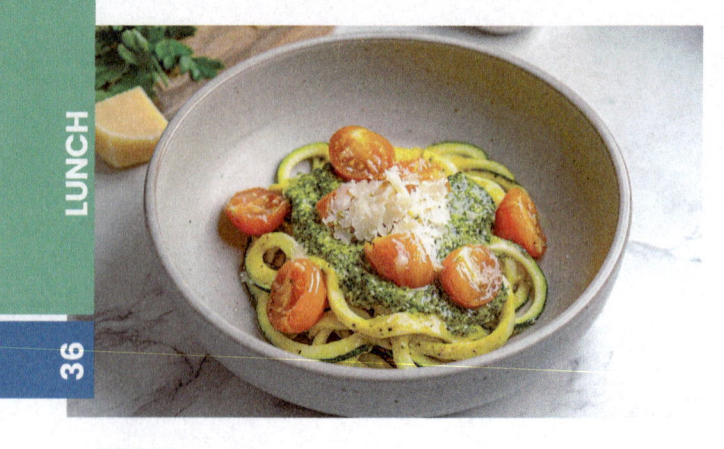

ZUCCHINI NOODLES WITH HOMEMADE DASH PESTO

Servings: 4
Prep Time: 15 minutes
Cook Time: 5 minutes

Nutrition Facts (per serving):
- Calories: 175
- Carbs: 11g
- Fat: 12g
- Fiber: 3g
- Sodium: 130mg
- Protein: 5g

INGREDIENTS:
- 4 medium zucchinis (about 600 g)
- 1 tablespoon olive oil (15 ml)
- 1 cup cherry tomatoes (150 g)
- 3 tablespoons homemade DASH pesto
- 2 tablespoons grated reduced-fat Parmesan cheese (optional)
- Pepper to taste (optional)
- 1 cup fresh basil leaves (packed)
- 2 tablespoons olive oil (30 ml)
- 2 tablespoons walnuts or sunflower seeds (20 g)
- 1 tablespoon lemon juice (15 ml)
- 1 tablespoon grated reduced-fat Parmesan cheese (optional)

INSTRUCTIONS:
1. Spiralize the zucchinis using a spiralizer or julienne peeler. Halve the cherry tomatoes.
2. Heat olive oil in a large skillet over medium heat. Add the zucchini noodles and cherry tomatoes. Sauté for 3–4 minutes, until the zucchini softens slightly but remains firm.
3. Remove from heat and stir in the DASH pesto until evenly coated.
4. Serve warm, topped with extra Parmesan if desired.

COLORFUL SHRIMP & AVOCADO BOWL

Servings: 15
Prep Time: 10 minutes
Cook Time: 4 minutes

Nutrition Facts (per serving):
- Calories: 350
- Carbs: 24g
- Fat: 14g
- Fiber: 6g
- Sodium: 220mg
- Protein: 28g

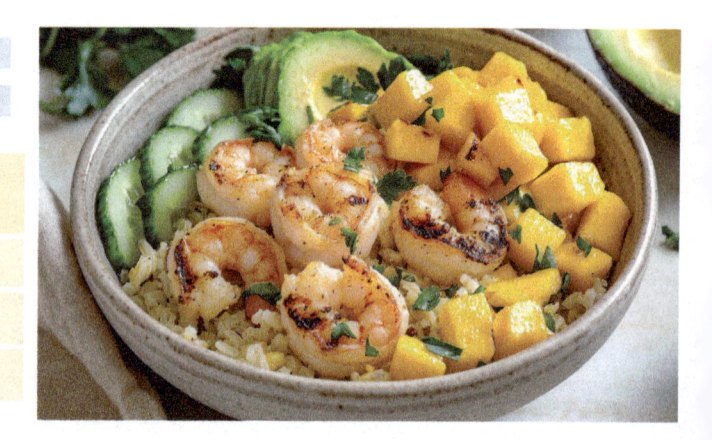

INGREDIENTS:
- 300 g shrimp, peeled and deveined
- 1 ripe avocado (150 g)
- 1 cup cooked brown rice (200 g)
- 1 cup mixed greens (50 g)
- 1/2 cup cucumber (75 g)
- 1 mango (150 g)
- 1/2 cup cooked corn kernels (75 g)
- 1 tablespoon olive oil (15 ml)
- 1 tablespoon lemon juice (5 ml)
- 1 teaspoon paprika (1 g)

INSTRUCTIONS:
1. Grill the shrimp with a bit of olive oil and paprika for 3–4 minutes per side, until cooked through.
2. In a large bowl, combine the cooked brown rice, avocado, mixed greens, cucumber, mango, corn, and grilled shrimp.
3. Drizzle with olive oil and lemon juice. Toss to combine.
4. Garnish with fresh parsley, if desired, and serve.

SAVORY TURKEY & VEGGIE LETTUCE WRAPS

Servings: 4
Prep Time: 15 minutes
Cook Time: 12 minutes

Nutrition Facts (per serving):
- Calories: 290
- Carbs: 8g
- Protein: 11 g
- Fiber: 2g
- Carbs: 32 g
- Protein: 25g

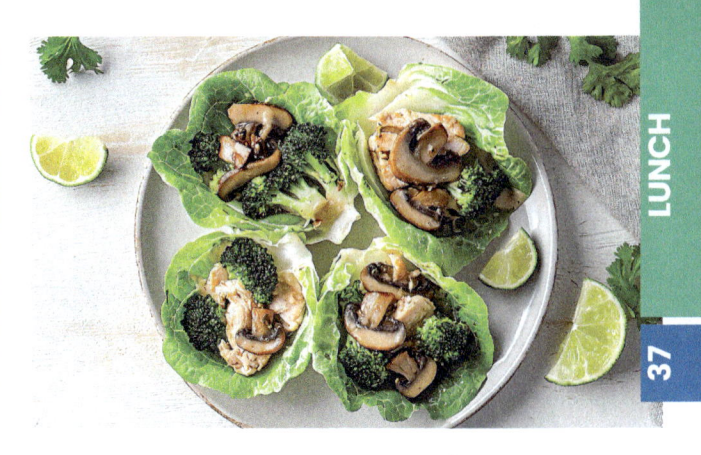

INGREDIENTS:

- 300 g turkey
- 1 small head of broccoli (about 100 g)
- 8–10 medium mushrooms (about 120 g)
- 1 tablespoon olive oil (15 ml)
- 2 tablespoons low-sodium soy sauce (30 ml)
- Juice of ½ lime
- Ground pepper to taste (optional)
- 8 large soft lettuce leaves (like butter or Bibb lettuce)

INSTRUCTIONS:

1. Dice the turkey into small bite-sized pieces. Clean and chop the mushrooms and broccoli into small, even pieces.
2. Heat the olive oil in a large skillet over medium heat. Add the turkey and cook for about 6–7 minutes, stirring occasionally, until fully cooked and lightly browned.
3. Add the chopped mushrooms and broccoli. Sauté for 5 more minutes until the vegetables are tender and any excess liquid has evaporated.
4. Stir in the soy sauce, lime juice, and a pinch of pepper. Mix well and remove from heat.
5. Rinse and dry the lettuce leaves. Spoon the filling into each leaf and serve as wraps or folded tacos.

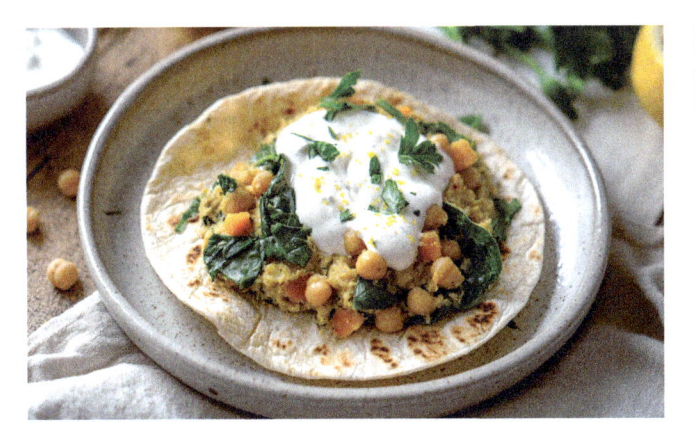

CHICKPEA & SPINACH WRAPS WITH CREAMY YOGURT SAUCE

Servings: 4
Prep Time: 10 minutes
Cook Time: 10 minutes

Nutrition Facts (per serving):
- Calories: 290
- Carbs: 32g
- Fat: 12g
- Fiber: 7g
- Sodium: 220mg
- Protein: 11g

INGREDIENTS:

- 1 tablespoon olive oil (15 ml)
- 1 can low-sodium chickpeas, drained and rinsed (15 oz / 425 g)
- 1 garlic clove (3 g)
- 1 small carrot (60 g)
- 2 cups fresh spinach (60 g)
- ½ teaspoon ground cumin (1 g)
- Black pepper to taste
- ½ cup plain Greek yogurt (120 g)
- Juice and Zest of ½ lemon
- 4 whole grain wraps or tortillas

INSTRUCTIONS:

1. Mince the garlic, dice the carrot, and roughly chop the spinach.
2. Heat olive oil in a skillet over medium heat. Sauté the garlic for 1 minute.
3. Add the chickpeas, grated carrot, cumin, and black pepper. Cook for 5–6 minutes, gently mashing some of the chickpeas with the back of a spoon.
4. Stir in the chopped spinach and cook for 2 more minutes, until wilted.
5. In a bowl, whisk the yogurt, lemon juice and lemon zest to create the sauce.
6. Warm the wraps, fill each with the chickpea mixture, and drizzle with the yogurt sauce before serving.

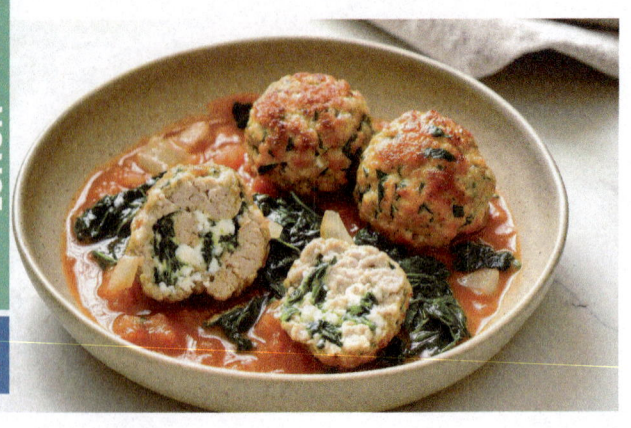

STUFFED TURKEY MEATBALLS WITH SPINACH & TOMATO

Servings: 4
Prep Time: 10 minutes
Cook Time: 20 minutes

Nutrition Facts (per serving):

Calories: 280	Fat: 13 g
Protein: 30 g	Fiber: 2 g
Carbs: 10 g	Sodium: 140 mg

INGREDIENTS:
- 1 lb ground turkey (450 g)
- 1 egg
- ¼ cup plain breadcrumbs (30 g)
- 1 tablespoon olive oil (15 ml)
- 1 teaspoon garlic powder (2 g)
- 1 teaspoon dried oregano (1 g)
- 1 ½ cups fresh spinach (45 g)
- 1 ½ cups no-salt-added crushed tomatoes (360 ml)
- 1 small onion (100 g)
- Black pepper to taste

INSTRUCTIONS:
1. Preheat the oven to 375°F (190°C).
2. In a skillet, sauté the chopped onion in olive oil for 3–4 minutes until soft. Add the spinach and cook for 1–2 minutes until wilted. Set aside to cool slightly.
3. In a large bowl, combine ground turkey, egg, breadcrumbs, garlic powder, oregano, pepper, and half of the sautéed onion-spinach mix. Mix until just combined.
4. Shape the mixture into small meatballs.
5. Place the meatballs in a baking dish. Pour the crushed tomatoes and the remaining spinach mixture around them.
6. Bake for about 18–20 minutes, or until the meatballs are cooked through. Serve warm and enjoy!

WHOLE WHEAT PASTA WITH SAUTÉED VEGGIES

Servings: 4
Prep Time: 15 minutes
Cook Time: 20 minutes

Nutrition Facts (per serving):

Calories: 300	Carbs: 53g
Fat: 7g	Fiber: 6g
Sodium: 150mg	Protein: 14g

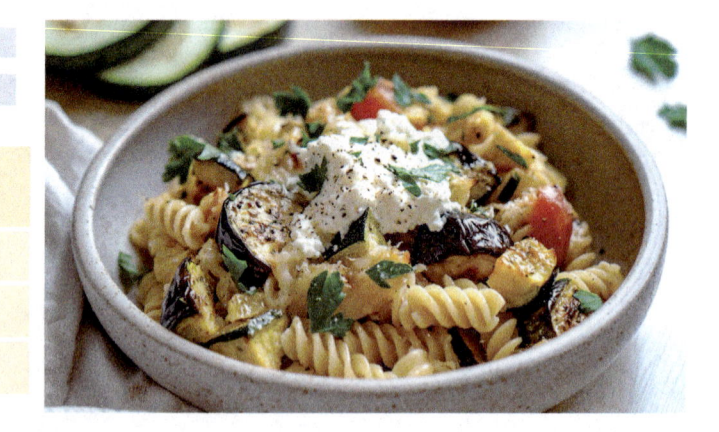

INGREDIENTS:
- 300 g whole wheat pasta
- 1 zucchini, sliced (150 g)
- 1 eggplant, diced (200 g)
- 1 tomato, diced (150 g)
- 1 cup low-fat cottage cheese (240 g)
- 1 tablespoon olive oil (15 ml) or olive oil spray
- 1 teaspoon dried oregano (1 g)
- 1/2 teaspoon garlic powder (1 g)
- Black pepper to taste
- 1/4 cup light cheese (optional)

INSTRUCTIONS:
1. Cook the whole wheat pasta according to package instructions. Drain and set aside.
2. Heat the olive oil in a large nonstick skillet over medium heat. Add the zucchini, eggplant, and tomato. Season with oregano, garlic powder, and black pepper. Cook, stirring occasionally, for 10–12 minutes until the vegetables are tender and lightly browned.
3. Once the vegetables are cooked, add the cooked pasta to the skillet and toss to combine.
4. Stir in the cottage cheese and cook for another 2–3 minutes until warmed through.
5. Serve the pasta with a sprinkle of light cheese on top (if desired) and garnish with fresh parsley.

SHAKSHUKA WITH SPINACH & BELL PEPPERS

Servings: 4
Prep Time: 10 minutes
Cook Time: 20 minutes

Nutrition Facts (per serving):
- Calories: 210
- Fat: 14g
- Sodium: 250mg
- Carbs: 10g
- Fiber: 4g
- Protein: 12g

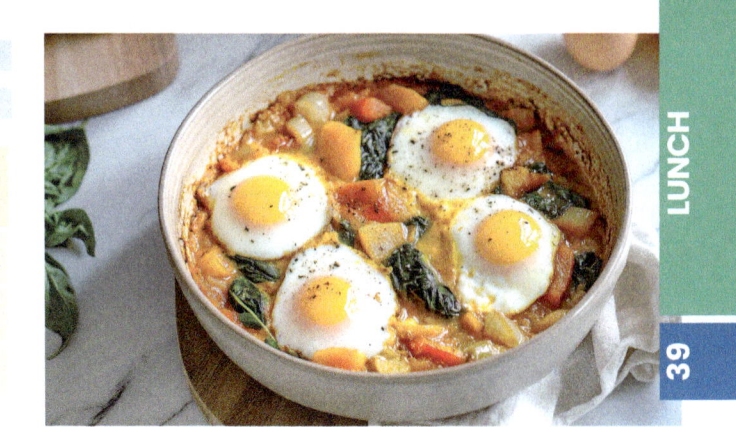

INGREDIENTS:
- 1 tablespoon olive oil (15 ml)
- 1 red bell pepper (120 g)
- 1 yellow bell pepper (120 g)
- 1 onion (100 g)
- 2 garlic cloves (3 g)
- 2 cups spinach (60 g)
- 4 large eggs
- 1 can (400 g) low-sodium diced tomatoes
- 1 teaspoon ground cumin (1 g)
- 1/2 teaspoon smoked paprika (1 g)
- Black pepper to taste
- 1/4 cup light cheese (optional)

INSTRUCTIONS:
1. Cut the bell peppers into strips, chop the onion, and mince the garlic.
2. Heat the olive oil in a large nonstick skillet over medium heat. Add the bell peppers, onion, and garlic. Cook for 5–7 minutes until the vegetables are soft.
3. Add the cumin, smoked paprika, and black pepper. Stir to coat the vegetables with the spices.
4. Add the diced tomatoes and spinach. Cook for another 5 minutes, until the spinach wilts and the sauce thickens.
5. Make four wells in the tomato mixture and crack an egg into each well. Cover the skillet and cook for 6–8 minutes, or until the eggs are cooked to your liking.
6. If desired, sprinkle the eggs with light cheese and let it melt for a minute before serving.

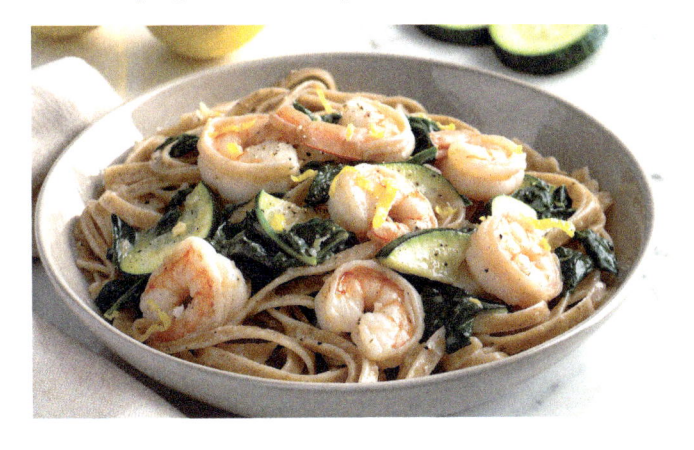

CREAMY LEMON FETTUCCINE WITH SHRIMP

Servings: 4
Prep Time: 10 minutes
Cook Time: 15 minutes

Nutrition Facts (per serving):
- Calories: 360
- Protein: 26 g
- Carbs: 35 g
- Fiber: 6 g
- Total Fat: 14 g
- Sodium: 230 mg

INGREDIENTS:
- 180 g whole wheat fettuccine
- 200 g raw shrimp
- 1 small zucchini (120 g)
- 2 cups fresh spinach (60 g)
- 1 tablespoon olive oil (15 ml)
- Juice and zest of 1 lemon
- ½ cup plain low-fat Greek yogurt (120 g)
- 1 garlic clove
- Black pepper to taste

INSTRUCTIONS:
1. Cook the fettuccine in boiling water as directed. Drain and set aside, reserving ¼ cup of cooking water.
2. In a large nonstick skillet over medium heat, heat the oil and cook the shrimp for 2–3 minutes per side, until pink. Remove and set aside.
3. Cut the zucchini into half-moons. Sauté for 3–4 minutes. Add spinach and cook until wilted.
4. Add the minced garlic, lemon zest, and juice. Stir in Greek yogurt and reserved pasta water to make a creamy sauce (do not boil).
5. Return the shrimp and pasta to the skillet and toss to combine.
6. Serve immediately and enjoy!

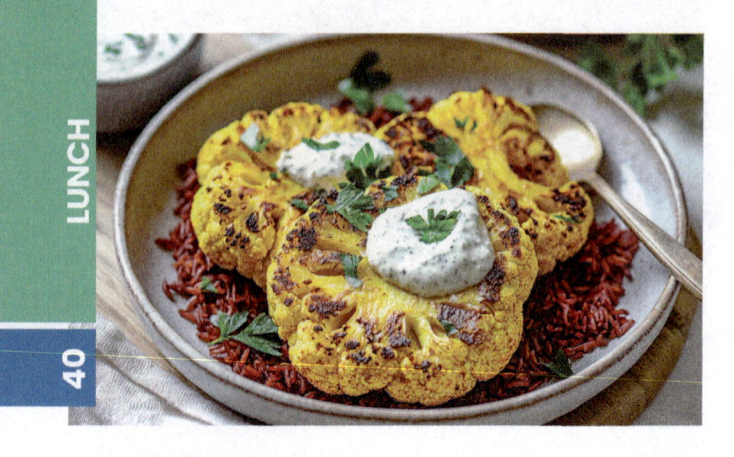

CURRIED CAULIFLOWER STEAKS WITH RED RICE & TZATZIKI

Servings: 4
Prep Time: 10 minutes
Cook Time: 30 minutes

Nutrition Facts (per serving):

Calories: 330	Fiber: 6 g
Protein: 9 g	Total Fat: 12 g
Carbs: 45 g	Sodium: 100 mg

INGREDIENTS:

- 2 medium cauliflower heads (approx. 1.2 kg)
- 1 cup red rice (180 g)
- 2 tablespoons olive oil (30 ml)
- 2 teaspoons curry powder (4 g)
- 1 teaspoon garlic powder (2 g)
- ½ teaspoon ground cumin (1 g)
- Black pepper to taste
- ½ cup DASH Tzatziki Sauce (120 g)
- Fresh parsley (optional, for garnish)

INSTRUCTIONS:

1. Preheat the oven to 400°F (200°C). Slice the cauliflower into thick "steaks" (2–3 cm).
2. In a small bowl, mix the olive oil with curry, garlic powder, cumin, and pepper. Brush over both sides of the cauliflower.
3. Place on a lined baking sheet and roast for 25–30 minutes, flipping halfway through, until golden and tender.
4. Meanwhile, rinse and cook the red rice according to package instructions.
5. Divide the cooked rice between 4 plates, top with the roasted cauliflower steaks, and spoon over the DASH Tzatziki Sauce.
6. Garnish with fresh parsley if desired.

SALMON & COUSCOUS SALAD WITH FRESH GREENS

Servings: 4
Prep Time: 10 minutes
Cook Time: 10 minutes

Nutrition Facts (per serving):

Calories: 370	Fiber: 4 g
Protein: 28 g	Total Fat: 18 g
Carbs: 26 g	Sodium: 90 mg

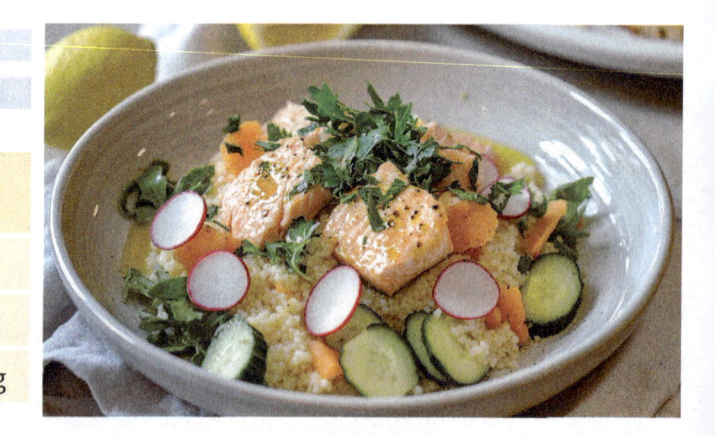

INGREDIENTS:

- 2 salmon fillets (approx. 360–400 g total)
- 1 ½ cups whole wheat couscous (240 g)
- 2 cups arugula or baby greens (60 g)
- 1 cucumber (150 g)
- 1 medium carrot (100 g)
- 5–6 radishes (60 g)
- 2 tablespoons olive oil (30 ml)
- 1 tablespoon lemon juice (15 ml)
- 1 tablespoon fresh parsley (optional)
- Black pepper to taste

INSTRUCTIONS:

1. Cook the couscous according to package instructions. Fluff with a fork and let cool.
2. Season the salmon with black pepper and cook in a nonstick skillet over medium heat for 3–4 minutes per side, until just cooked through.
3. Meanwhile, slice the radishes, grate the carrot, and chop the cucumber.
4. In a large bowl, combine the couscous, arugula, carrot, cucumber, and radishes.
5. Flake the salmon into bite-sized pieces and gently toss into the salad.
6. Drizzle with olive oil and lemon juice. Garnish with finely chopped fresh parsley if using.

DINNER

*Wind down with warm, comforting meals that love your heart.
Easy dinners that bring joy to your plate—without the pressure.*

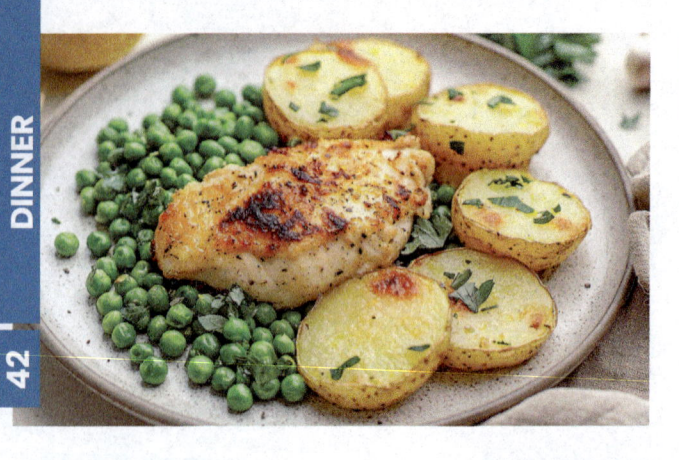

LEMON & GARLIC CHICKEN WITH SAUTÉED VEGGIES

Servings: 4
Prep Time: 15 minutes
Cook Time: 20 minutes

Nutrition Facts (per serving):

Calories: 250	Carbs: 18g
Fat: 11g	Fiber: 5g
Sodium: 120mg	Protein: 24g

INGREDIENTS:

- 4 boneless, skinless chicken breasts (400 g)
- 2 tablespoons olive oil (30 ml) or olive oil spray
- 1 lemon (juice and zest)
- 2 garlic cloves
- 1 teaspoon dried oregano (1 g)
- ¼ teaspoon ground black pepper
- 2 medium potatoes (300 g)
- 1/2 cup peas (75 g)

INSTRUCTIONS:

1. Season the chicken breasts with black pepper, oregano, lemon zest, and minced garlic. Squeeze half of the lemon juice over the chicken. Let it marinate for 5–10 minutes.
2. Heat 1 tablespoon of olive oil in a large nonstick skillet over medium heat. Add the chicken breasts and cook for 6–7 minutes per side, until golden brown and fully cooked through.
3. Remove the chicken and set aside. In the same skillet, add the remaining olive oil. Add the potatoes and sauté for 6–7 minutes until tender and slightly golden.
4. Add the peas to the skillet and continue to sauté for 2–3 minutes until tender.
5. Return the chicken to the pan and drizzle with the remaining lemon juice.
6. Cook for an additional 2 minutes to combine flavors and serve with the sautéed veggies.

SPICED LENTIL PATTIES WITH FRESH SALAD

Servings: 2
Prep Time: 5 minutes
Cook Time: 5 minutes

Nutrition Facts (per serving):

Calories: 270	Fiber: 8 g
Protein: 13 g	Fat: 12 g
Carbs: 27 g	Sodium: 120 mg

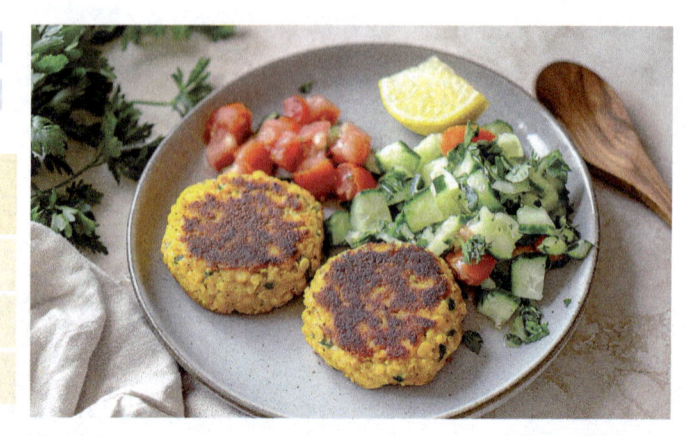

INGREDIENTS:

- 1 cup cooked lentils (200 g)
- ½ cup rolled oats (40 g)
- 1 small carrot (60 g)
- 1 small onion (70 g)
- 1 egg
- 1 tablespoon olive oil (15 ml)
- 1 teaspoon cumin
- ¼ teaspoon ground black pepper
- 2 medium tomatoes (240 g)
- ½ cucumber (100 g)
- Juice of ½ lemon

INSTRUCTIONS:

1. Grate the carrot and finely chop the onion. In a bowl, mix with lentils, oats, egg, cumin, and pepper.
2. Mash slightly until a chunky dough forms. Shape into 8 small patties.
3. Heat olive oil in a skillet over medium heat and cook patties for 3–4 minutes per side until golden.
4. Meanwhile, dice the tomatoes into small chunks and chop the cucumber. Toss with lemon juice to make a quick salad.
5. Serve 2 patties per person with a generous spoonful of fresh salad.
6. Enjoy your meal.

FRESH FISH WITH A COLORFUL VEGGIE MEDLEY

Servings: 4
Prep Time: 15 minutes
Cook Time: 25 minutes

Nutrition Facts (per serving):
- Calories: 210
- Fat: 9g
- Sodium: 80mg
- Carbs: 8g
- Fiber: 3g
- Protein: 24g

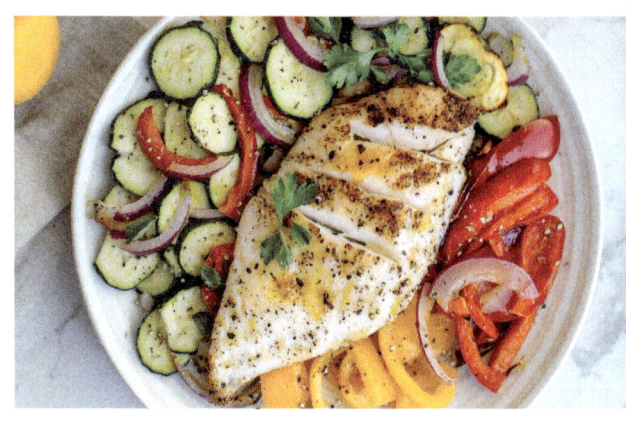

INGREDIENTS:
- 4 white fish fillets (cod or hake) (500 g)
- 1 zucchini (150 g)
- 1 red bell pepper (120 g)
- 1 yellow bell pepper (120 g)
- 1/2 red onion (60 g)
- Juice of 1 orange (40 ml)
- 2 tablespoons olive oil (30 ml) or olive oil spray
- 1 teaspoon dried oregano (1 g)
- Black pepper to taste
- Fresh parsley for garnish (optional)

INSTRUCTIONS:
1. Wash the vegetables. Slice the zucchini and bell peppers into thin strips. Slice the red onion.
2. Lightly coat a large nonstick skillet with olive oil spray and place over medium heat. Add the vegetables and sauté for 8–10 minutes until slightly tender.
3. Push the vegetables to the sides of the skillet and place the fish fillets in the center. Season with black pepper and oregano.
4. Cover the skillet with a lid, then pour the orange juice over the fish. Reduce heat to low and cook for 10–12 minutes, or until the fish is opaque and flakes easily with a fork.
5. Remove from heat and let sit for 2 minutes with the lid on.
6. Serve the fish over the warm vegetables and garnish with chopped parsley if desired.

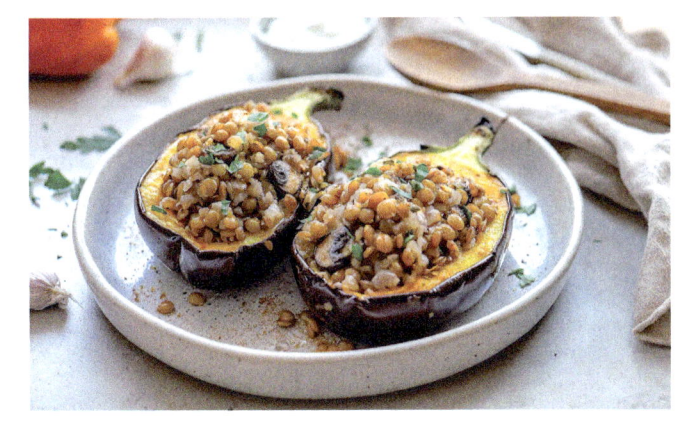

EGGPLANTS WITH TASTY LENTILS & MUSHROOMS

Servings: 4
Prep Time: 15 minutes
Cook Time: 30 minutes

Nutrition Facts (per serving):
- Calories: 230
- Protein: 10 g
- Carbs: 25 g
- Fat: 10 g
- Fiber: 9 g
- Sodium: 90 mg

INGREDIENTS:
- 2 medium eggplants (about 500 g)
- 1 cup cooked lentils (160 g)
- 1 cup mushrooms (90 g)
- 1 tablespoon olive oil (15 ml)
- 1 small onion (100 g)
- 2 garlic cloves (6 g)
- ½ teaspoon dried thyme (1 g)
- Black pepper to taste
- ¼ teaspoon smoked paprika (0.5 g)

INSTRUCTIONS:
1. Preheat the oven to 400°F (200°C). Slice the eggplants in half lengthwise and scoop out the flesh, leaving a 1 cm border. Place the halves on a baking tray and roast for 20 minutes.
2. Finely chop the onion, garlic, and eggplant flesh. Slice the mushrooms for added texture.
3. In a skillet, heat the olive oil. Sauté the onion and garlic for 2–3 minutes. Add mushrooms and chopped eggplant flesh. Cook until tender, about 6–7 minutes.
4. Stir in the cooked lentils, thyme, paprika, and black pepper. Cook for 2 more minutes to combine.
5. Spoon the mixture into the roasted eggplant halves and return to the oven for another 10 minutes. Serve warm and enjoy.

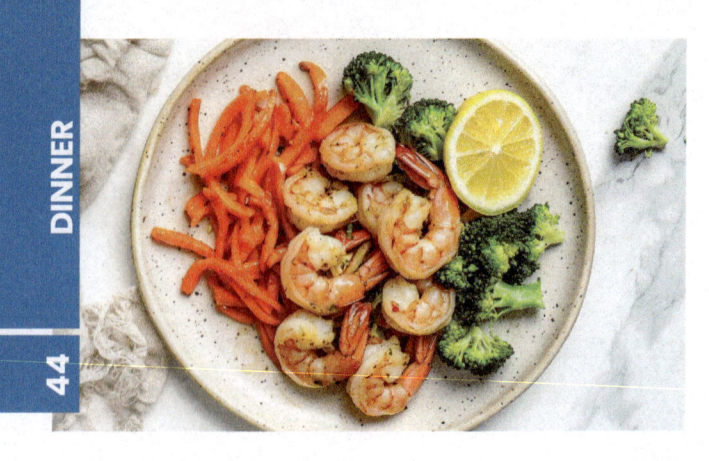

SHRIMP STIR-FRY WITH COLORFUL VEGGIES

Servings: 4
Prep Time: 10 minutes
Cook Time: 12 minutes

Nutrition Facts (per serving):

Calories: 248	Fiber: 2 g
Protein: 27 g	Fat: 11 g
Carbs: 10 g	Sodium: 268 mg

INGREDIENTS:

- 1 tablespoon olive oil (15 ml)
- 1 pound raw shrimp, peeled and deveined (450 g)
- 1 red bell pepper (120 g)
- 1 medium carrot (80 g)
- 1 cup broccoli florets (90 g)
- 2 garlic cloves (6 g)
- 1 tablespoon low-sodium soy sauce (15 ml)
- Juice of ½ lemon

INSTRUCTIONS:

1. Thinly slice the bell pepper and carrot into thin strips. Cut the broccoli into small florets. Mince the garlic.
2. Heat olive oil in a large nonstick skillet over medium-high heat.
3. Add the garlic and shrimp. Cook for 2-3 minutes until the shrimp turn pink. Remove and set aside.
4. In the same skillet, add bell pepper, carrot, and broccoli. Stir-fry for 5-6 minutes until just tender.
5. Return the shrimp to the pan. Add the soy sauce and lemon juice. Stir well and cook for 1-2 more minutes.
6. Serve warm. Garnish with a lemon wedge if desired. Enjoy your meal.

HEALTHY TURKEY & SPINACH LASAGNA

Servings: 4
Prep Time: 20 minutes
Cook Time: 30 minutes

Nutrition Facts (per serving):

Calories: 315	Carbs: 26g
Fat: 13g	Fiber: 4g
Sodium: 140mg	Protein: 25g

INGREDIENTS:

- 6 whole wheat lasagna sheets (120 g)
- 200 g ground turkey (lean, min. 93%)
- 1 cup fresh spinach (30 g)
- 1 cup unsalted crushed tomatoes (240 g)
- 1/2 cup low-sodium ricotta cheese (125 g)
- 1 tablespoon low-fat milk (15 ml)
- 1 small onion (50 g)
- 1 garlic clove (3 g)
- 1 tablespoon olive oil (15 ml)
- 1 teaspoon dried oregano (1 g)
- 1/2 teaspoon dried basil (0.5 g)
- Black pepper to taste

INSTRUCTIONS:

1. Cook the lasagna noodles according to package directions. Drain and set aside.
2. Peel and chop the onion. Peel and mince the garlic. Wash and chop the spinach.
3. In a skillet, heat the olive oil over medium heat. Add the onion and garlic, and sauté for 3-4 minutes. Add the ground turkey, breaking it apart as it cooks, until fully browned. Stir in the crushed tomatoes, spinach, basil, oregano, and black pepper. Simmer for 5-6 minutes.
4. In a bowl, mix the ricotta. Add the milk only if the texture is too thick to spread.
5. In a small baking dish, layer: a spoonful of turkey mixture, then noodles, ricotta, and repeat until finished. Top with the remaining turkey mixture and, if desired, sprinkle with shredded cheese.
6. Cover with foil and bake at 180°C (350°F) for 20-25 minutes. Uncover and bake 5 more minutes to brown the top. Let cool slightly before serving.

SALMON WITH HERBED YOGURT & ROASTED VEGGIES

Servings: 4
Prep Time: 10 minutes
Cook Time: 20 minutes

Nutrition Facts (per serving):

Calories: 340	Carbs: 15g
Fat: 18g	Fiber: 4g
Sodium: 105mg	Protein: 33g

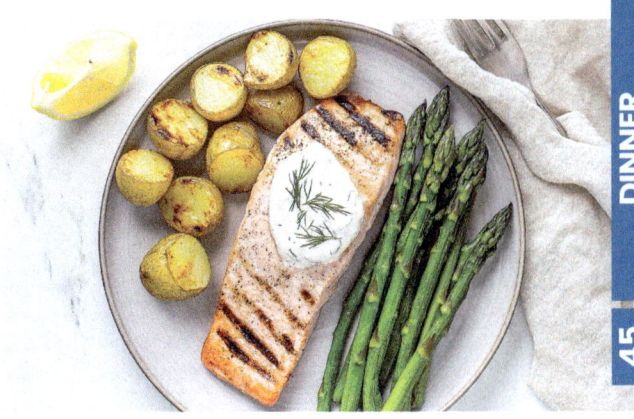

INGREDIENTS:
- 4 salmon fillets (approx. 150 g each)
- 450 g baby potatoes
- 400 g asparagus spears
- 1 tablespoon olive oil (15 ml)
- 1 tablespoon lemon juice (15 ml)
- 1 teaspoon lemon zest
- 1 cup plain low-fat Greek yogurt (240 g)
- 1 tablespoon fresh dill (optional)
- Black pepper to taste

INSTRUCTIONS:
1. Preheat the oven to 400°F (200°C). Cut the baby potatoes in half and place them on a baking tray. Drizzle with half the olive oil and season with pepper. Roast for 10 minutes.
2. Trim the asparagus and add them to the tray with the potatoes. Drizzle with the remaining olive oil and return to the oven for another 10–12 minutes, or until golden and tender.
3. Heat a grill pan over medium-high heat. Brush the salmon fillets with lemon juice and season with pepper. Grill for 4–5 minutes per side, or until cooked through and nicely charred.
4. While the salmon cooks, finely chop the dill. In a small bowl, mix the yogurt with dill, lemon zest, and a pinch of pepper.
5. Serve each salmon fillet with a spoonful of herbed yogurt on top, accompanied by roasted potatoes and asparagus.

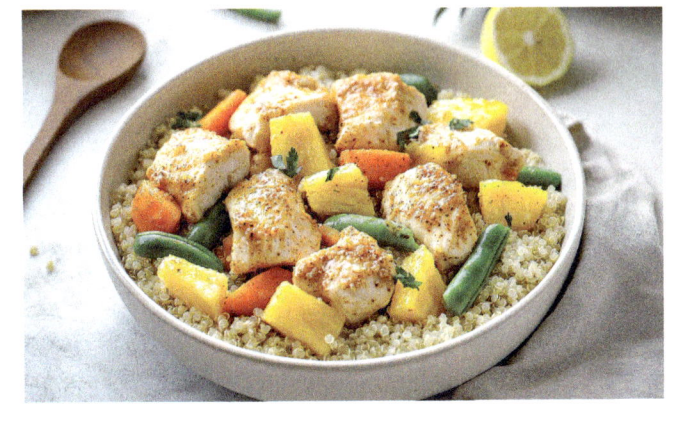

LIGHT TROPICAL CHICKEN CURRY

Servings: 4
Prep Time: 10 minutes
Cook Time: 20 minutes

Nutrition Facts (per serving):

Calories: 285	Fiber: 5 g
Protein: 24 g	Total Fat: 10 g
Carbs: 28 g	Sodium: 150 mg

INGREDIENTS:
- 1 chicken breast (200 g)
- 1 cup fresh pineapple chunks (165 g)
- 1 cup green beans (100 g)
- 1 medium carrot (60 g)
- 1 small onion (80 g)
- 1 tablespoon olive oil (15 ml)
- 1 teaspoon mild curry powder (2 g)
- ½ teaspoon turmeric (1 g)
- Black pepper to taste
- ½ cup low-sodium vegetable broth or water (120 ml)
- 1 cup cooked brown rice or quinoa, to serve (185 g)

INSTRUCTIONS:
1. Peel and slice the carrot. Chop the onion. Cut the green beans and dice the chicken into small cubes.
2. Heat olive oil in a large skillet over medium heat. Sauté the onion and carrot for 3–4 minutes.
3. Add the chicken and cook for 5–6 minutes, stirring occasionally until browned.
4. Stir in curry powder, turmeric, and pepper. Mix well to coat everything evenly.
5. Add pineapple chunks, green beans, and broth or water. Cover and simmer for 8–10 minutes, until the chicken is cooked through and veggies are tender.
6. Serve warm over brown rice or quinoa.

DINNER

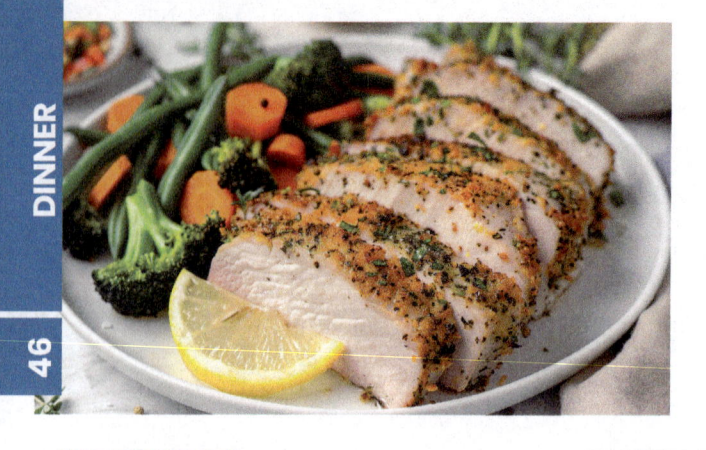

TENDER HERB-CRUSTED PORK WITH GARDEN VEGGIES

Servings: 4
Prep Time: 15 minutes
Cook Time: 25 minutes

Nutrition Facts (per serving):

Calories: 240	Carbs: 10g
Fat: 11g	Fiber: 4g
Sodium: 95mg	Protein: 26g

INGREDIENTS:
- 4 pork loin medallions (360–400 g total), trimmed
- 2 cups broccoli florets (200 g)
- 1 cup sliced carrots (120 g)
- 1 cup green beans (120 g)
- 2 tablespoons olive oil (30 ml) or olive oil spray
- 2 teaspoons dried thyme (2 g)
- 1 teaspoon garlic powder (2 g)
- 2 teaspoon lemon juice (10 ml)
- Black pepper to taste

INSTRUCTIONS:
1. Wash and cut the vegetables. Trim the pork and pat it dry with paper towel.
2. In a small bowl, mix the thyme, garlic powder, and black pepper. Rub the seasoning evenly over both sides of each pork medallion.
3. Heat 1 tablespoon of olive oil in a nonstick skillet or shallow casserole over medium heat. Sear the pork for 3–4 minutes per side until lightly browned. Remove and set aside.
4. In the same pan, add the remaining oil and sauté the broccoli, carrots, and green beans for 6–7 minutes.
5. Return the pork to the pan, add the lemon juice, and cover with a lid. Reduce heat to low and cook for 10 more minutes, or until the pork is fully cooked and the vegetables are tender.
6. Let rest 2 minutes before serving.

HAKE "EN PAPILLOTE" WITH LEMON, ZUCCHINI & EGGPLANT

Servings: 4
Prep Time: 10 minutes
Cook Time: 20 minutes

Nutrition Facts (per serving):

Calories: 215	Fiber: 3 g
Protein: 27 g	Total Fat: 9 g
Carbs: 8 g	Sodium: 95 mg

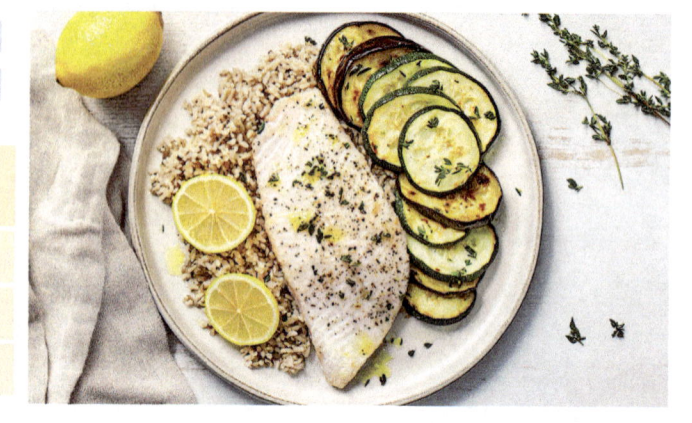

INGREDIENTS:
- 4 hake fillets (about 5 oz / 140 g each)
- 1 medium zucchini (120 g)
- ½ medium eggplant (150 g)
- 1 lemon (120 g)
- 1 tablespoon olive oil (15 ml)
- 1 teaspoon dried thyme (1 g)
- Black pepper to taste
- 1 cup cooked brown rice (200 g), optional

INSTRUCTIONS:
1. Preheat the oven to 400°F (200°C). Cut the zucchini and eggplant into thin rounds. Slice the lemon into thin rounds.
2. Cut 4 large squares of parchment paper. Place one hake fillet in the center of each.
3. Top each fillet with zucchini, eggplant, and a few thin lemon slices for flavor.
4. Drizzle with olive oil, sprinkle with thyme and pepper to taste.
5. Fold the paper over the fish and seal the edges tightly to create a packet.
6. Bake for 10–15 minutes, or until the fish flakes easily with a fork. Remove the parchment before serving, and plate with brown rice if desired.

BAKED CHICKEN WITH APPLE & MASHED CAULIFLOWER

Servings: 4
Prep Time: 10 minutes
Cook Time: 30 minutes

Nutrition Facts (per serving):
- Calories: 264
- Protein: 26 g
- Carbs: 14 g
- Fiber: 4 g
- Total Fat: 11 g
- Sodium: 115 mg

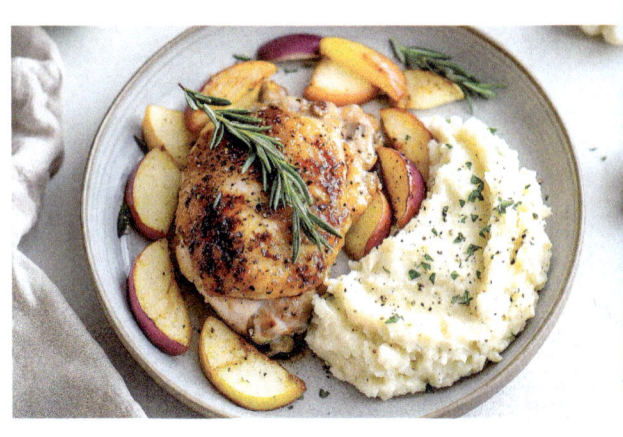

INGREDIENTS:
- 4 boneless skinless chicken thighs (about 500 g)
- 2 apples (300 g)
- 1 tablespoon olive oil (15 ml)
- ½ teaspoon garlic powder (1.5 g)
- 1 teaspoon dried rosemary (1 g)
- Black pepper to taste
- ½ head of cauliflower (300 g)
- 2–3 tablespoons unsweetened plant-based milk (30–45 ml)
- A pinch of ground nutmeg

INSTRUCTIONS:
1. Preheat the oven to 400°F (200°C). Slice the apple. Cut cauliflower into florets.
2. Place chicken and apple slices in a baking dish. In a small bowl, mix olive oil, garlic powder, rosemary, and pepper.
3. Pour the mixture over the chicken and toss to coat evenly.
4. On a separate tray, add the cauliflower florets and lightly spray or drizzle with oil.
5. Bake both trays for 30 minutes, until chicken is golden and cauliflower is tender.
6. Blend the cauliflower with plant-based milk and nutmeg until smooth. Serve with the baked chicken and apple mixture.

WARM & RUSTIC BEEF STEW

Servings: 4
Prep Time: 15 minutes
Cook Time: 40 minutes

Nutrition Facts (per serving):
- Calories: 305
- Protein: 28 g
- Carbs: 18 g
- Fiber: 4 g
- Total Fat: 14 g
- Sodium: 190 mg

INGREDIENTS:
- 2 medium carrots (150 g)
- 1 ½ cups mushrooms (120 g)
- 1 medium potato (150 g)
- 12 oz lean beef stew meat (340 g)
- 1 tablespoon olive oil (15 ml)
- 1 small onion (100 g)
- 2 garlic cloves (6 g)
- 1 tablespoon tomato paste (15 g)
- 2 cups low-sodium beef broth (480 ml)
- ½ teaspoon dried thyme (0.5 g)
- ¼ teaspoon ground ginger (0.5 g)
- Black pepper to taste

INSTRUCTIONS:
1. Peel and chop all the vegetables. Mince the garlic and cut the beef into cubes if needed.
2. In a large pot, heat olive oil over medium heat. Sauté the onion and garlic for 2–3 minutes.
3. Add the beef and brown on all sides, about 5–6 minutes.
4. Stir in tomato paste and cook 1 minute. Add carrots, mushrooms, potato, broth, thyme, ginger, and pepper.
5. Bring to a gentle boil and stir to combine the flavors before covering.
6. Reduce heat to low, cover, and simmer 30 minutes until beef is tender. Garnish with parsley if desired and serve.

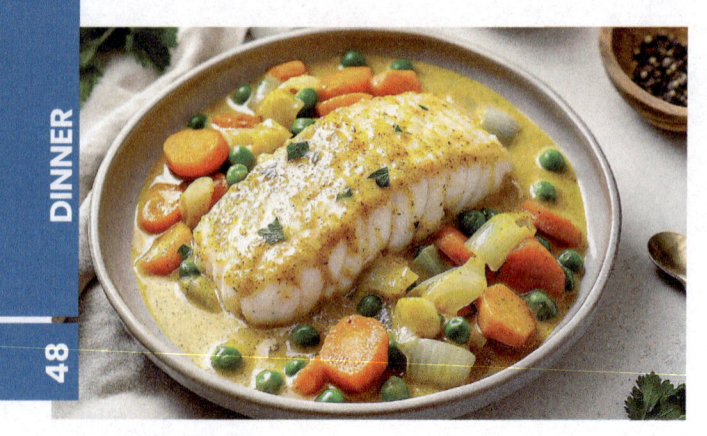

GENTLE COD CURRY WITH VEGGIES

Servings: 4
Prep Time: 10 minutes
Cook Time: 15 minutes

Nutrition Facts (per serving):

Calories: 220	Fiber: 3 g
Protein: 26 g	Total Fat: 10 g
Carbs: 8 g	Sodium: 105 mg

INGREDIENTS:
- 4 cod fillets (about 500 g total)
- 1 cup green peas (140 g)
- 1 medium carrot (120 g)
- 1 small leek (60 g)
- 2 tablespoons low-fat plain yogurt (30 g)
- 1 tablespoon olive oil (15 ml)
- 1 teaspoon curry powder (2 g)
- 1 teaspoon turmeric (2 g)
- ½ teaspoon ground cumin (1 g)
- ½ teaspoon garlic powder (1 g)
- 1 tablespoon lemon juice (15 ml)

INSTRUCTIONS:
1. Wash the vegetables. Peel and slice the carrot into rounds. Slice the leek into rings.
2. In a non-stick pan, heat the olive oil over medium heat. Add the leek and carrot, and sauté for 3–4 minutes until slightly tender.
3. Add the curry powder, turmeric, cumin, garlic powder, and black pepper. Stir well to coat the vegetables with the spices.
4. Place the cod fillets on top. Cover with a lid and cook over low heat for 7–8 minutes, until the fish is opaque and flakes easily.
5. Remove from heat. Add the yogurt and lemon juice. Gently stir everything together to create a smooth, mild curry sauce that coats the fish and vegetables.
6. Serve warm, garnished with fresh cilantro if desired.

PORK TENDERLOIN WITH FENNEL SAUCE

Servings: 4
Prep Time: 15 minutes
Cook Time: 30 minutes

Nutrition Facts (per serving):

Calories: 305	Sodium: 95mg
Total Fat: 11g	Potassium: 670mg
Saturated Fat: 2.5g	Fiber: 3g

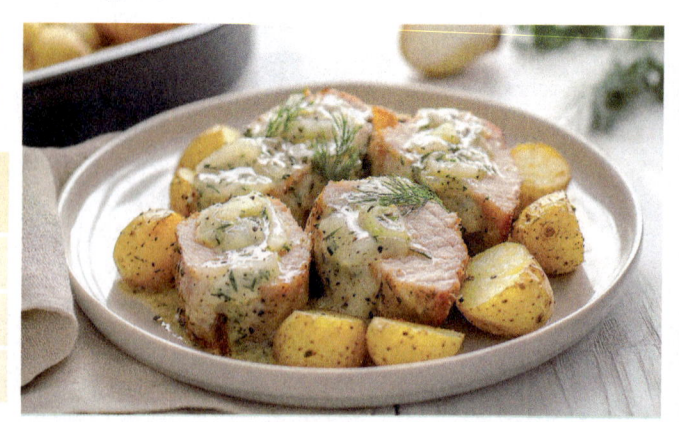

INGREDIENTS:
- 400 g pork tenderloin, trimmed
- 1 tablespoon olive oil (15 ml) or olive oil spray
- 1 fennel bulb (200 g)
- ½ small onion (25 g)
- 1 garlic clove (3 g)
- ½ cup unsalted low-sodium vegetable broth (120 ml)
- 1 teaspoon dried thyme (1 g)
- 1 teaspoon lemon juice (5 ml)
- 300 g baby potatoes
- Black pepper to tase

INSTRUCTIONS:
1. Preheat oven to 190°C (375°F). Halve the baby potatoes, toss with oil spray and pepper, and roast for 30 minutes, flipping halfway.
2. Trim the pork, season with pepper and thyme.
3. Sear the pork in a hot skillet with olive oil for 5–6 minutes until golden.
4. Transfer to a baking dish and roast 15–20 minutes, until it reaches 63°C (145°F). Rest 5 minutes before slicing.
5. Meanwhile, slice the fennel and onion, and mince the garlic. Sauté in the same skillet for 5 minutes. Add broth and lemon juice, cover, and simmer 8–10 minutes.
6. Serve sliced pork over roasted potatoes, topped with fennel sauce and fronds if desired.

COZY WHITE BEAN STEW WITH A TWIST

Servings: 4
Prep Time: 10 minutes
Cook Time: 25 minutes

Nutrition Facts (per serving):
Calories: 220 | Protein: 9 g
Carbs: 28 g | Fat: 7 g
Fiber: 8 g | Sodium: 180 mg

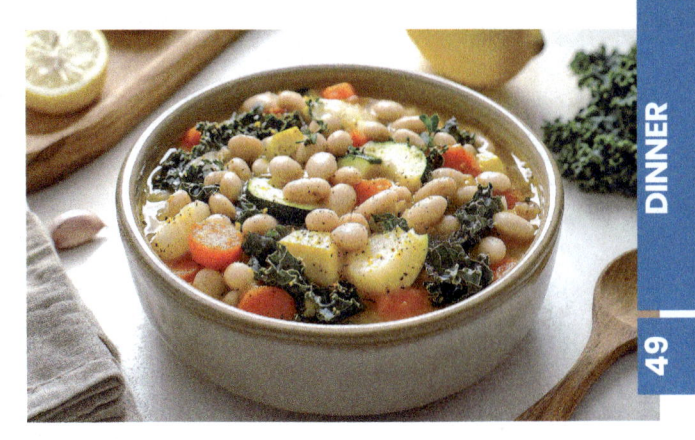

INGREDIENTS:

- 2 medium carrots (120 g)
- 1 medium zucchini (150 g)
- 1 can no-salt-added white beans, drained and rinsed (15 oz / 425 g)
- 3 cups chopped kale (90 g)
- 1 tablespoon olive oil (15 ml)
- 1 small onion (80 g)
- 2 garlic cloves (6 g)
- 1 teaspoon ground ginger (2 g)
- ½ teaspoon ground turmeric (1 g)
- 3 cups low-sodium vegetable broth (720 ml)
- Juice of ½ lemon

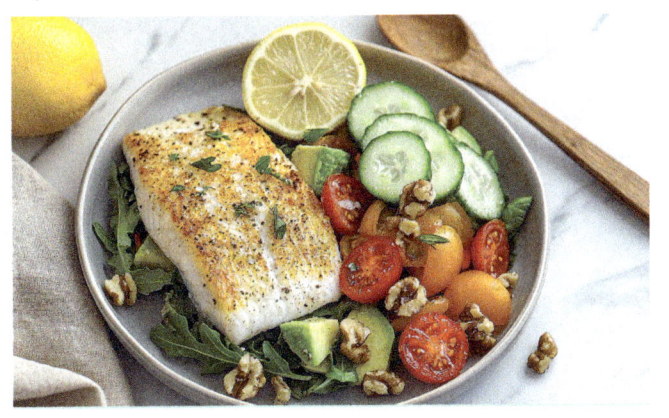

INSTRUCTIONS:

1. Dice the onion and peel and slice the carrots. Mince the garlic and slice the zucchini.
2. In a large pot, heat olive oil over medium heat. Add the onion and garlic and sauté for 3–4 minutes.
3. Stir in the ginger and turmeric, cooking for 1 minute to release their aroma.
4. Add the carrots and zucchini and cook for 5 minutes, stirring occasionally.
5. Pour in the broth and add the beans. Bring to a gentle boil, then reduce heat and simmer for 10 minutes.
6. Stir in the kale and simmer for 5 more minutes, until tender but still vibrant. Finish with a squeeze of lemon and serve warm.

TILAPIA WITH FRESH GARDEN SALAD & LEMON VINAIGRETTE

Servings: 4
Prep Time: 10 minutes
Cook Time: 10 minutes

Nutrition Facts (per serving):
Calories: 240 | Carbs: 40g
Fat: 4g | Fiber: 7g
Sodium: 60mg | Protein: 9g

INGREDIENTS:

- 4 tilapia fillets (500 g)
- 2 tablespoons lemon juice (30 ml), divided
- 2 teaspoons ground coriander (4 g)
- 2 teaspoons olive oil (10 ml)
- 4 cups baby greens or arugula (120 g)
- 1 cup cherry tomatoes (150 g), halved
- 1 cucumber (120 g), sliced
- 1 avocado (120 g), thinly sliced
- 2 tablespoons chopped walnuts (20 g)
- • 2 teaspoons apple cider vinegar (10 ml)

INSTRUCTIONS:

1. Pat dry the tilapia fillets. Rub with lemon juice, coriander, and black pepper. Let rest for a few minutes.
2. Heat the olive oil in a non-stick skillet over medium heat. Cook the tilapia for 3–4 minutes per side, until golden and cooked through. Set aside.
3. While the fish cooks, halve the cherry tomatoes, slice the cucumber, and thinly slice the avocado.
4. In a large bowl, combine the baby greens, cherry tomatoes, cucumber, avocado, and chopped walnuts.
5. Drizzle with apple cider vinegar and lemon juice. Toss gently to coat.
6. Serve the fish over or alongside the fresh salad. Enjoy warm.

DINNER

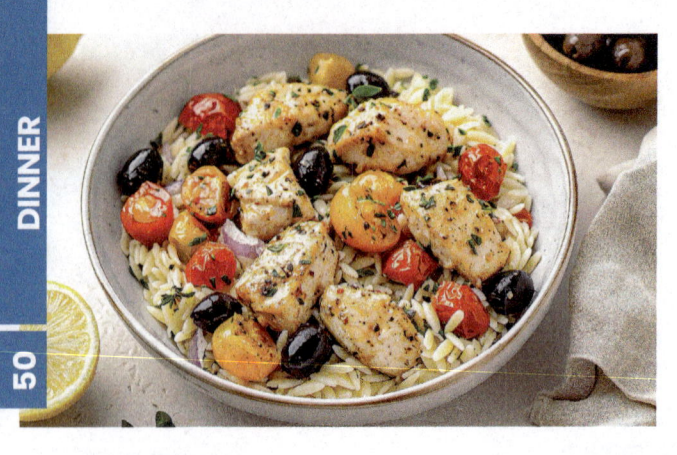

50

MEDITERRANEAN CHICKEN WITH ORZO & VEGGIES

Servings: 4

Prep Time: 10 minutes

Cook Time: 20 minutes

Nutrition Facts (per serving):

Calories: 310	Fiber: 3 g
Protein: 27 g	Total Fat: 10 g
Carbs: 28 g	Sodium: 220 mg

INGREDIENTS:

- 2 skinless chicken breasts (approx. 300 g)
- ¾ cup orzo pasta (120 g)
- 1 cup cherry tomatoes (150 g)
- ¼ cup pitted black olives (40 g)
- 2 tablespoons red onion (20 g)
- 1 teaspoon olive oil (5 ml)
- ½ teaspoon dried oregano (1 g)
- Black pepper to taste

INSTRUCTIONS:

1. Cook the orzo in a pot of boiling water according to package instructions. Drain and set aside.
2. Dice the chicken into medium chunks and season with oregano and black pepper. Slice the cherry tomatoes in half and finely chop the onion.
3. In a non-stick skillet, heat the olive oil over medium heat. Add the chicken and cook for 5–6 minutes, stirring occasionally, until golden and cooked through.
4. Add the red onion, tomatoes, and olives. Cook for 3–4 minutes until the tomatoes soften.
5. Add the cooked orzo and mix everything gently in the skillet.
6. Serve warm. For extra freshness, you can drizzle with a little lemon juice before serving.

ASIAN-STYLE GINGER TOFU & VEGGIE STIR-FRY

Servings: 4

Prep Time: 15 minutes

Cook Time: 12 minutes

Nutrition Facts (per serving):

Calories: 340	Fiber: 6 g
Protein: 17 g	Total Fat: 14 g
Carbs: 36 g	Sodium: 230 mg

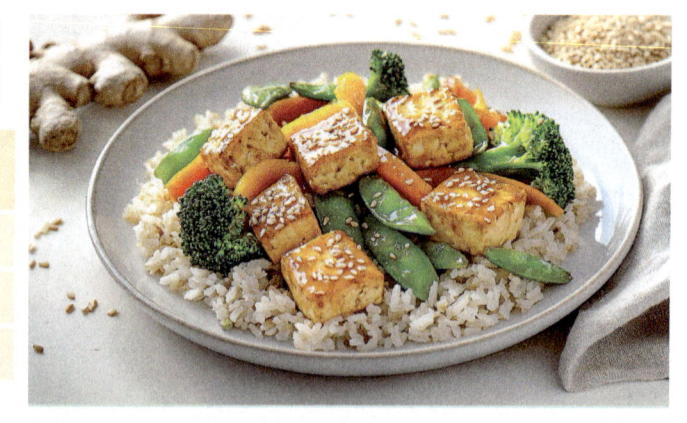

INGREDIENTS:

- 1 block firm tofu (approx. 350 g)
- 1 tablespoon olive oil (15 ml)
- 1½ cups broccoli florets (150 g)
- 1 large carrot (100 g)
- 1 cup snow peas or sugar snap peas (100 g)
- ½ cup yellow bell pepper (50 g)
- 2 garlic cloves (6 g)
- 1 tablespoon fresh ginger (10 g)
- 2 tablespoons low-sodium soy sauce (30 ml)
- 1 tablespoon rice vinegar (15 ml)
- 1 teaspoon sesame oil (5 ml) (optional)
- ½ teaspoon cornstarch + 2 tablespoons water (for thickening, optional)
- 2 cups cooked brown rice (300 g), for serving

INSTRUCTIONS:

1. Cut the tofu into cubes and pat dry with a paper towel to remove excess moisture.
2. In a non-stick skillet, heat olive oil over medium heat. Add the tofu and cook for 5–6 minutes, turning gently to brown on all sides. Remove and set aside.
3. Peel and slice the carrot. Mince the garlic, grate the ginger, and slice the bell pepper into strips.
4. In the same skillet, sauté the broccoli, carrot, snow peas, and bell pepper for about 4 minutes, until just tender but still crisp.
5. Return the tofu to the pan. Add garlic, ginger, soy sauce, vinegar, and sesame oil if using. Stir well and cook 2 more minutes. For a thicker sauce, stir in the cornstarch-water mix.
6. Serve over warm brown rice.

SNACKS & DRINKS

*Smart bites to fuel your day—no guilt, just goodness.
Healthy nibbles for when hunger strikes between meals.*

SNACKS & DRINKS

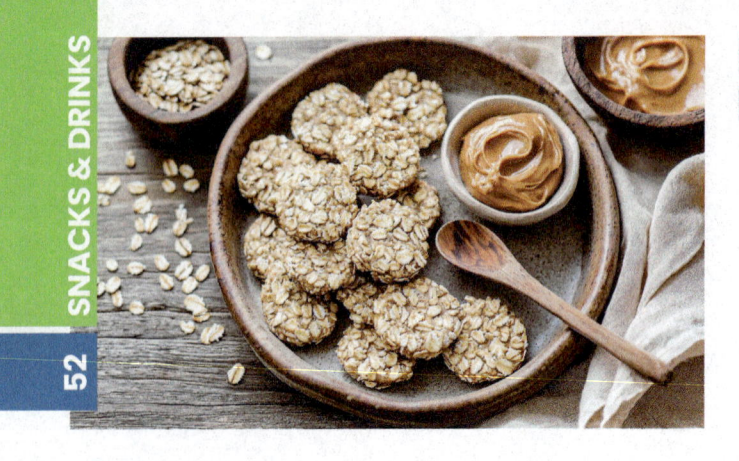

52

NO-BAKE OAT BITES WITH PEANUT BUTTER & SEEDS

Servings: 2
Prep Time: 10 minutes
Cook Time: —

Nutrition Facts (per serving):

Calories: 160	Carbs: 18g
Fat: 8g	Fiber: 3g
Sodium: 40mg	Protein: 4g

INGREDIENTS:

- ½ cup rolled oats (50 g)
- 1 tablespoon ground flaxseeds (8 g)
- ½ tablespoon unsalted, unsweetened peanut butter (8 g)
- 1 tablespoon nuts or seeds of choice (10 g)
- ½ tablespoon honey or maple syrup (7 g)
- 1 tablespoon unsweetened applesauce (15 g)
- ¼ teaspoon cinnamon (0.5 g)
- ½ teaspoon vanilla extract (2.5 ml)
- 2 tablespoons extra rolled oats (20 g), for coating

INSTRUCTIONS:

1. In a medium bowl, combine oats, ground flaxseeds, chopped nuts or seeds, and cinnamon.
2. In a small saucepan, warm the peanut butter, honey, applesauce, and vanilla over low heat until smooth.
3. Pour the warm mixture over the dry ingredients and stir until well combined.
4. With slightly damp hands, form small bite-sized balls. Roll each one in the extra oats to coat the surface.
5. Place on a plate and refrigerate for at least 30 minutes before serving.

CREAMY HUMMUS WITH ROASTED VEGGIE STICKS

Servings: 2
Prep Time: 10 minutes
Cook Time: 15 minutes

Nutrition Facts (per serving):

Calories: 240	Fiber: 7 g
Protein: 8 g	Total Fat: 11 g
Carbs: 26 g	Sodium: 140 mg

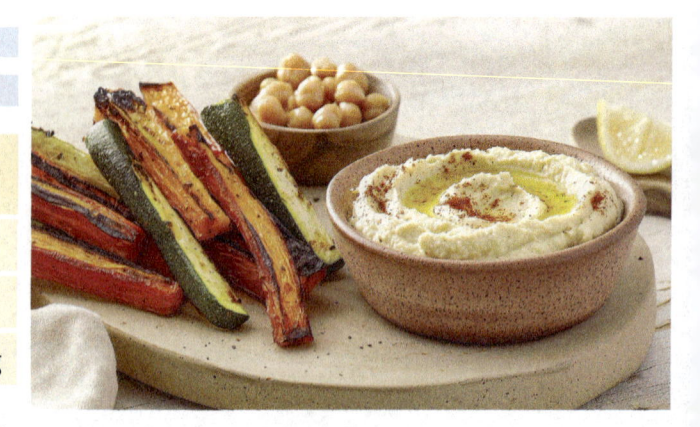

INGREDIENTS:

- 1 can low-sodium chickpeas, drained and rinsed (15 oz / 425 g)
- 1 tablespoon tahini (15 g)
- Juice of ½ lemon
- 1 small garlic clove (3 g)
- 1 tablespoon olive oil (15 ml)
- 1–2 tablespoons water, as needed
- 1 medium carrot (70 g)
- 1 small zucchini (120 g)
- ½ red bell pepper (60 g)
- ½ teaspoon dried oregano (1 g)
- ¼ teaspoon ground cumin (0.5 g)
- Black pepper to taste

INSTRUCTIONS:

1. Preheat the oven to 400°F (200°C). Line a baking tray with parchment paper.
2. Cut the carrot, zucchini, and bell pepper into sticks.
3. Place them on the tray, drizzle with half the olive oil, and season with oregano, cumin, and black pepper. Roast for 15 minutes, flipping halfway through.
4. Meanwhile, prepare the hummus: In a food processor, blend chickpeas, tahini, lemon juice, garlic, remaining olive oil, and 1 tablespoon of water until smooth. Add more water if needed for desired texture.
5. Transfer the hummus to a small bowl and serve with the warm roasted veggie sticks.
6. Optionally, drizzle with a little extra olive oil or a pinch of paprika for presentation.

DASH TZATZIKI SAUCE

Servings: 2
Prep Time: 10 minutes
Cook Time: —

Nutrition Facts (per serving):
Calories: 45 | Carbs: 3g
Fat: 1g | Fiber: 0g
Sodium: 30mg | Protein: 5g

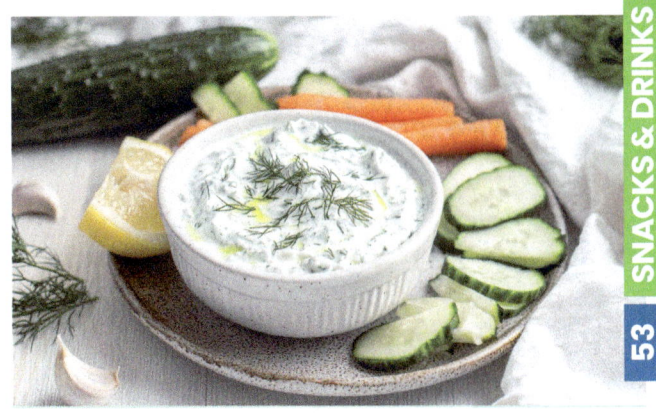

INGREDIENTS:
- ½ cup low-fat Greek yogurt (120 g)
- ¼ medium cucumber (approx. 50 g)
- ½ tablespoon fresh lemon juice (7 ml)
- ½ garlic clove, optional
- ½ tablespoon fresh dill (finely chopped) or ¼ teaspoon dried dill, optional
- Black pepper to taste

INSTRUCTIONS:
1. Peel and grate the cucumber. Squeeze excess liquid from the grated cucumber using a clean towel or paper towels.
2. In a bowl, combine the yogurt, grated cucumber, lemon juice, finely minced garlic (if using), dill, and pepper.
3. Mix until smooth and creamy.
4. Taste and adjust seasoning as needed.
5. Serve immediately or refrigerate until ready to use.

SERVING TIP:
Perfect as a dip with whole-grain pita, carrot sticks, or fresh veggies. Also great with grilled dishes!

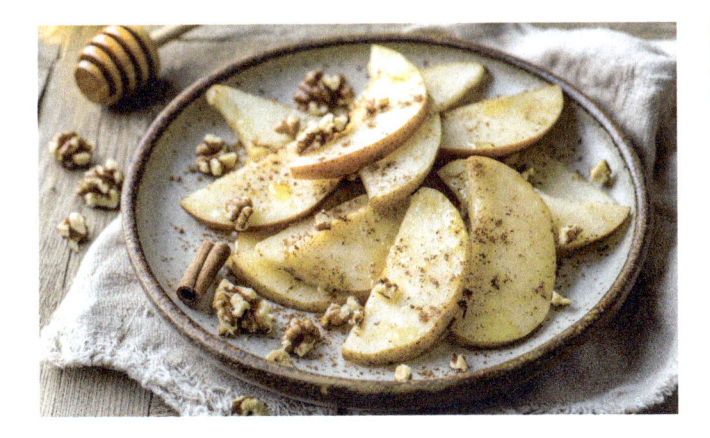

SWEET BAKED APPLE SLICES WITH A NUTTY TWIST

Servings: 2
Prep Time: 5 minutes
Cook Time: 15 minutes

Nutrition Facts (per serving):
Calories: 150 | Carbs: 22g
Fat: 7g | Fiber: 3g
Sodium: 2mg | Protein: 1g

INGREDIENTS:
- 2 medium apples (about 300 g)
- 1 teaspoon olive oil (5 ml)
- ½ teaspoon ground cinnamon (1 g)
- 1 tablespoon walnuts (7 g)
- Optional: 1 teaspoon honey or maple syrup (5 ml)

INSTRUCTIONS:
1. Preheat the oven to 375°F (190°C).
2. Core the apples and slice them into thin wedges.
3. In a bowl, toss the apple slices with olive oil and cinnamon until well coated.
4. Spread the slices on a parchment-lined baking sheet in a single layer.
5. Bake for 15 minutes, or until tender and slightly golden.
6. Sprinkle with chopped walnuts and drizzle with honey or maple syrup if using. Serve warm.

STORAGE TIP:
You can double the batch and keep leftovers in an airtight container in the fridge for up to 3 days.

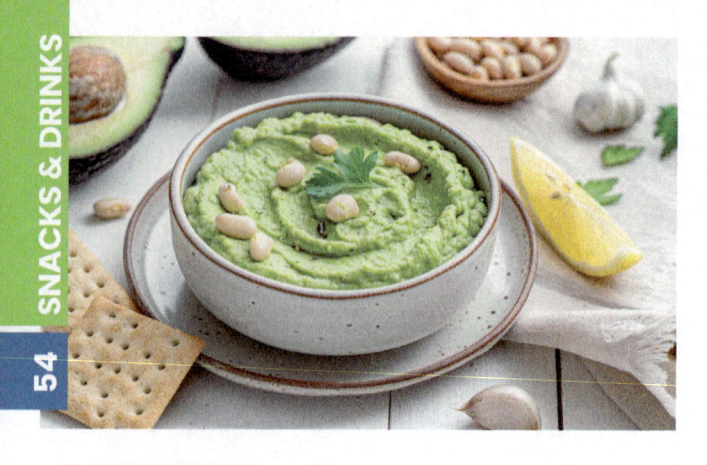

CREAMY AVOCADO & WHITE BEAN DIP

Servings: 2
Prep Time: 5 minutes
Cook Time: —

Nutrition Facts (per serving):

Calories: 210	Carbs: 16g
Fat: 15g	Fiber: 6g
Sodium: 80mg	Protein: 5g

INGREDIENTS:
- 1 ripe avocado (150 g)
- ½ cup canned white beans, drained and rinsed (130 g)
- Juice of ½ lemon
- ½ garlic clove (1.5 g)
- 1 tablespoon olive oil (15 ml)
- ¼ teaspoon ground cumin (0.5 g)
- Black pepper to taste
- Optional: fresh parsley or chives for garnish
- 8–10 whole grain crackers

INSTRUCTIONS:
1. In a bowl, mash the avocado and white beans together until mostly smooth (or use a food processor for a creamier texture).
2. Add lemon juice, grated garlic, olive oil, cumin, and pepper. Mix well until combined.
3. Transfer to a small serving bowl and garnish with herbs if desired.
4. Serve with whole grain crackers.

DID YOU KNOW?
Avocado and beans make a fiber-rich dip that's creamy, filling, and great for heart health.

SPICY DASH TRAIL MIX

Servings: 2
Prep Time: 5 minutes
Cook Time: —

Nutrition Facts (per serving):

Calories: 240	Carbs: 40g
Fat: 4g	Fiber: 7g
Sodium: 60mg	Protein: 9g

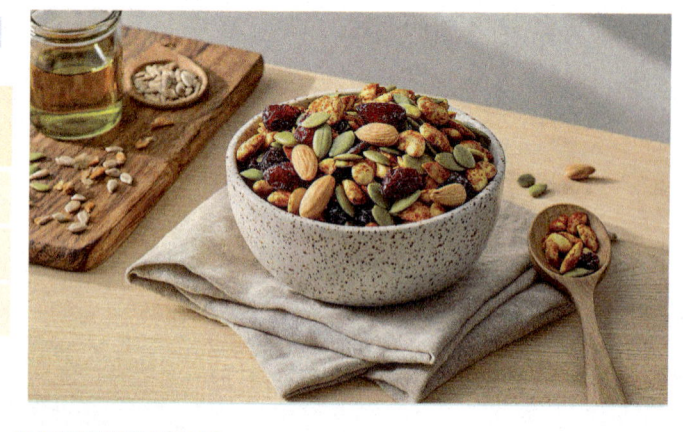

INGREDIENTS:
- 2 tablespoons unsalted almonds (18 g)
- 2 tablespoons unsalted cashews (18 g)
- 1 tablespoon pumpkin seeds (10 g)
- 1 tablespoon sunflower seeds (10 g)
- 1 tablespoon dried cranberries or raisins (10 g)
- ⅛ teaspoon smoked paprika (0.25 g)
- A pinch of cayenne pepper (optional)
- ¼ teaspoon olive oil (1.25 ml)

INSTRUCTIONS:
1. In a bowl, mix all the nuts and seeds with the dried fruit.
2. Drizzle with olive oil and sprinkle the paprika and cayenne pepper (if using).
3. Toss well to evenly coat.
4. Serve immediately or store in an airtight container for up to 5 days.

EXPERT TIP
Feel free to swap nuts or dried fruit based on what you have—just make sure they're unsalted and unsweetened.

MINI BAKED LENTIL FALAFELS WITH YOGURT-HERB DIP

Servings: 2
Prep Time: 15 minutes
Cook Time: 20 minutes

Nutrition Facts (per serving):
Calories: 260
Fat: 12g
Sodium: 110mg
Carbs: 28g
Fiber: 7g
Protein: 12g

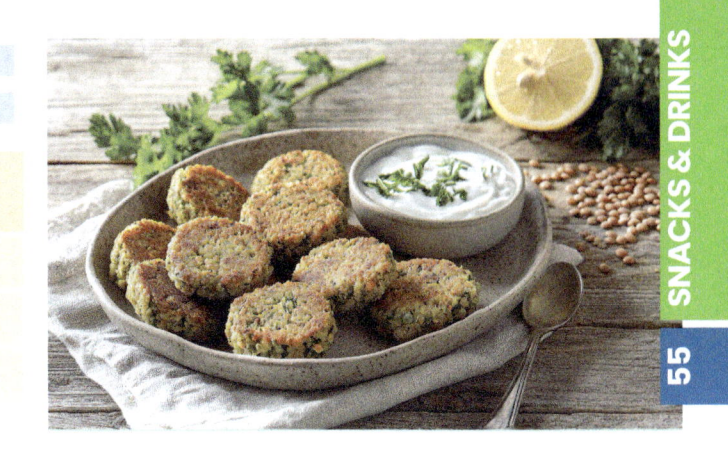

INGREDIENTS:
- ½ cup cooked lentils (100 g)
- ¼ cup rolled oats (20 g)
- 1 garlic clove (3 g)
- 1 small carrot (60 g)
- 1 tablespoon fresh parsley (3 g)
- ½ teaspoon ground cumin (1 g)
- ¼ teaspoon ground coriander (0.5 g)
- 1 tablespoon olive oil (15 ml)
- Black pepper to taste
- Cooking spray or extra olive oil for baking

For the Dip
- ½ cup plain Greek yogurt (120 g)
- 1 tablespoon lemon juice (15 ml)
- 1 tablespoon chopped fresh mint or parsley (3 g)
- Black pepper to taste

INSTRUCTIONS:
1. Preheat oven to 375°F (190°C). Line a baking tray with parchment paper.
2. In a food processor, combine lentils, oats, garlic, grated carrot, parsley, and spices. Pulse until a textured dough forms.
3. Shape the mixture into 8–10 small falafel balls and place them on the tray.
4. Lightly spray or brush the falafels with olive oil.
5. Bake for 18–20 minutes, flipping halfway, until golden and slightly crisp.
6. While baking, mix all dip ingredients in a bowl. Serve the warm falafels with the yogurt dip on the side.

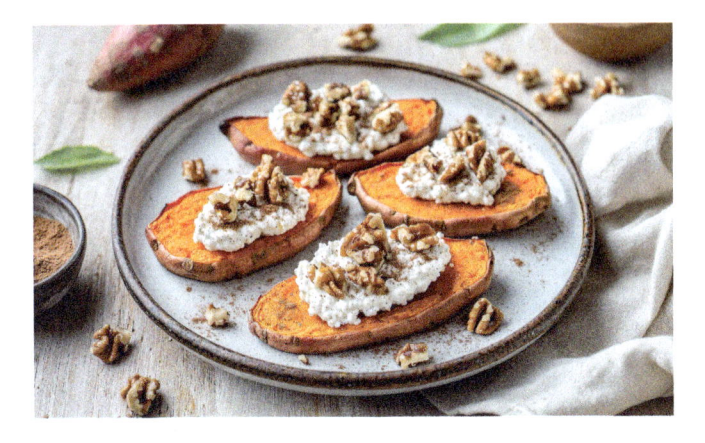

SWEET POTATO TOASTS WITH COTTAGE CHEESE & WALNUTS

Servings: 2
Prep Time: 10 minutes
Cook Time: 20 minutes

Nutrition Facts (per serving):
Calories: 190
Protein: 10 g
Carbs: 22 g
Fiber: 4 g
Total Fat: 8 g
Sodium: 125 mg

INGREDIENTS:
- 1 medium sweet potato (250 g)
- ½ cup low-fat cottage cheese (small curd, 120 g)
- 2 tablespoons walnuts (15 g)
- ¼ teaspoon ground cinnamon (optional)
- Olive oil spray

INSTRUCTIONS:
1. Preheat the oven to 400°F (200°C).
2. Slice the sweet potato lengthwise into ½-inch thick slices.
3. Lightly spray both sides with olive oil and place on a baking sheet.
4. Bake for 20 minutes, flipping halfway, until tender and lightly crisped.
5. Let cool slightly, then top each slice with cottage cheese, chopped walnuts, and a pinch of cinnamon if desired.
6. Serve warm or at room temperature.

DID YOU KNOW?
Sweet potato toasts are a great alternative to bread—nutritious, satisfying, and naturally gluten-free.

CRUNCHY SEED CRACKERS WITH HERBS

Servings: 2 (makes about 8 small crackers)
Prep Time: 10 minutes
Cook Time: 25–30 min.

Nutrition Facts (per serving):

Calories: 160	Fiber: 5 g
Protein: 5 g	Total Fat: 13 g
Carbs: 7 g	Sodium: 25 mg

INGREDIENTS:
- 2 tablespoons chia seeds (20 g)
- 2 tablespoons flaxseeds (whole or ground) (17 g)
- 2 tablespoons sesame seeds (18 g)
- 2 tablespoons sunflower seeds (17 g)
- ¼ teaspoon dried rosemary or thyme (0.5 g)
- ⅛ teaspoon garlic powder (0.25 g)
- Black pepper to taste
- ¼ cup water (60 ml)
- Olive oil spray (optional)

INSTRUCTIONS:
1. Preheat the oven to 160°C (320°F) and line a baking tray with parchment paper.
2. In a bowl, mix all seeds with herbs, garlic powder, and pepper.
3. Add the water and stir well. Let the mixture sit for about 10 minutes, until it thickens.
4. Spread the mixture evenly onto the baking sheet, flattening it with a spatula to about 3–4 mm thick.
5. Lightly spray with olive oil (optional) and bake for 25–30 minutes, flipping halfway if needed, until golden and crisp.
6. Let cool completely before breaking into pieces.

CITRUSY DASH GUACAMOLE

Servings: 2
Prep Time: 10 minutes
Cook Time: —

Nutrition Facts (per serving):

Calories: 140	Carbs: 8g
Fat: 11g	Fiber: 5g
Sodium: 10mg	Protein: 2g

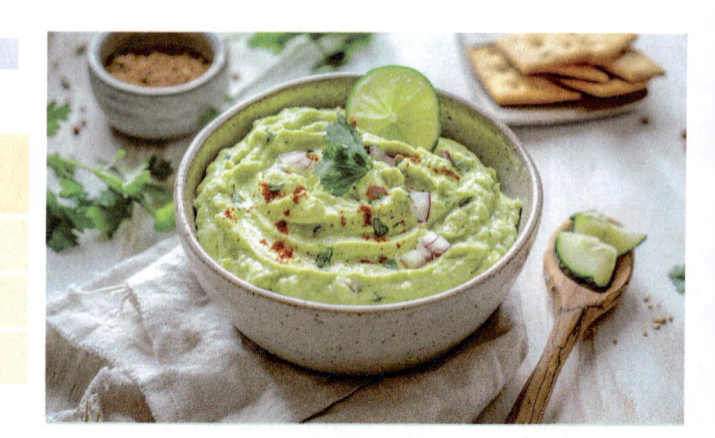

INGREDIENTS:
- 1 ripe avocado (approx. 125 g)
- Juice of ½ lime
- ½ small tomato (40 g)
- ½ tablespoon red onion (5 g)
- 1 tablespoon fresh cilantro (optional)
- ⅛ teaspoon ground cumin
- Black pepper to taste
- Ground paprika, for garnish (optional)

INSTRUCTIONS:
1. Cut the avocados in half, remove the pits, and scoop the flesh into a bowl.
2. Mash with a fork until smooth or slightly chunky, depending on your preference.
3. Dice the tomato and finely chop the onion. Stir both into the avocado along with lime juice, cumin, and black pepper.
4. Add finely chopped fresh cilantro if desired, and mix until well combined.
5. Garnish with extra cilantro and a pinch of paprika for color, if desired.
6. Serve immediately with whole-grain crackers or raw veggie sticks.

DASH-FRIENDLY POPCORN

Servings: 2
Prep Time: 5 minutes
Cook Time: 5 minutes

Nutrition Facts (per serving):
- Calories: 110
- Fat: 6g
- Sodium: 50mg
- Carbs: 13g
- Fiber: 2g
- Protein: 2g

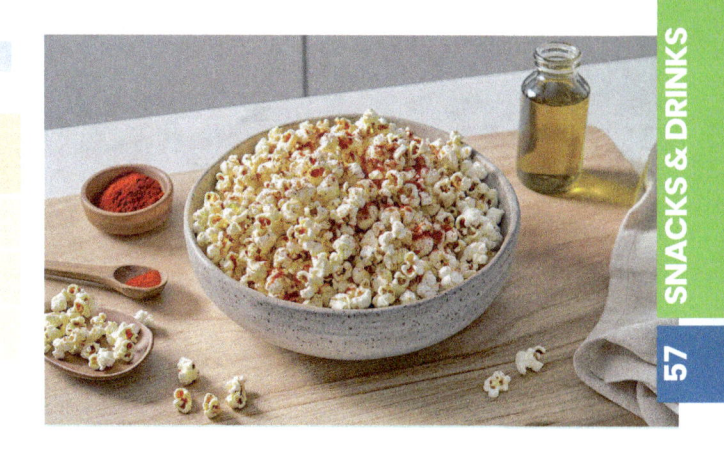

INGREDIENTS:
- ¼ cup popcorn kernels (45 g)
- 1½ teaspoons olive oil (7 ml)
- ½ teaspoon sweet paprika (1 g)

INSTRUCTIONS:
1. Heat the olive oil in a large pot over medium heat.
2. Add the popcorn kernels and cover with a lid.
3. Shake the pot occasionally as the kernels pop, keeping the lid slightly ajar to release steam.
4. When the popping slows down, remove from heat and let it sit for 30 seconds to finish popping.
5. Sprinkle with paprika (and optional garlic powder or herbs), toss well, and enjoy warm.

FLAVOR TIP:
Skip the butter and salt—olive oil and spices give this snack all the flavor, without the extra sodium.

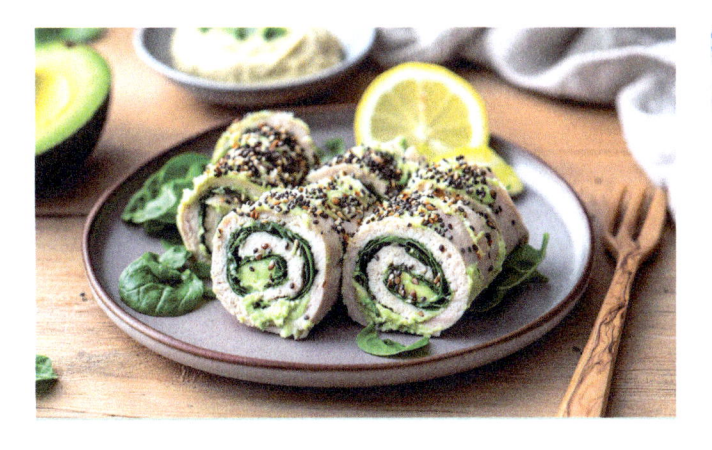

SAVORY ROLL-UPS WITH TURKEY, AVOCADO & SPINACH

Servings: 2 (makes 6 bite-sized roll-ups)
Prep Time: 10 minutes
Cook Time: —

Nutrition Facts (per serving):
- Calories: 240
- Fat: 4g
- Sodium: 60mg
- Carbs: 40g
- Fiber: 7g
- Protein: 9g

INGREDIENTS:
- 4 slices no-salt-added turkey breast (120 g)
- ½ ripe avocado (60 g)
- 1 handful fresh spinach or arugula (20 g)
- 1 teaspoon lemon juice (5 ml)
- Ground black pepper, to taste
- Mixed seeds (e.g. sesame, chia, flax), optional for garnish

INSTRUCTIONS:
1. Mash the avocado in a small bowl with lemon juice and a pinch of pepper.
2. Lay the turkey slices flat on a clean surface.
3. Spread a thin layer of mashed avocado on each slice.
4. Add a few spinach or arugula leaves.
5. Roll up each slice tightly and place seam side down.
6. Sprinkle with mixed seeds for extra texture and visual appeal.
7. Cut each roll into two bite-sized pieces for easier serving and a more elegant presentation, just like sushi rolls.

EXPERT TIP:
If the roll-ups don't stay closed easily, use a toothpick to hold them together until serving.

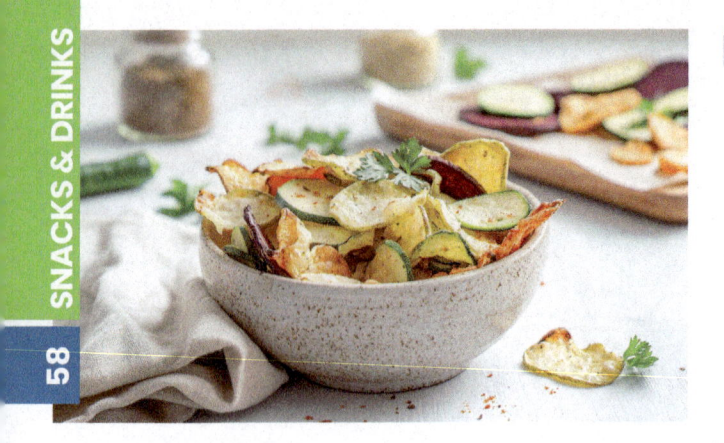

HOMEMADE BAKED VEGGIE CHIPS

Servings: 2
Prep Time: 10 minutes
Cook Time: 25 minutes

Nutrition Facts (per serving):

Calories: 110	Fiber: 3 g
Protein: 2 g	Total Fat: 5 g
Carbs: 16 g	Sodium: 70 mg

INGREDIENTS:
- 1 small sweet potato (150 g)
- 1 small beet (100 g)
- 1 small zucchini (120 g)
- 1 tablespoon olive oil (15 ml)
- ¼ teaspoon paprika (0.5 g)
- ¼ teaspoon garlic powder (0.5 g)
- Black pepper to taste

INSTRUCTIONS:
1. Preheat the oven to 180°C (350°F) and line a baking tray with parchment paper.
2. Wash the vegetables and thinly slice them using a sharp knife or mandoline.
3. In a large bowl, toss the veggie slices with olive oil, paprika, garlic powder, and black pepper.
4. Arrange the slices in a single layer on the prepared tray, making sure they don't overlap.
5. Bake for 20–25 minutes, flipping halfway through, until crisp and golden.
6. Let them cool slightly before serving for maximum crunch.

EXPERT TIP:
Slice your veggies super thin for the crispiest chips. Mix colors for a fun and tasty result.

GREEN REVITALIZING SMOOTHIE

Servings: 2
Prep Time: 5 minutes
Cook Time: —

Nutrition Facts (per serving):

Calories: 140	Fiber: 4 g
Protein: 2.5 g	Total Fat: 2.5 g
Carbs: 30 g	Sodium: 55 mg

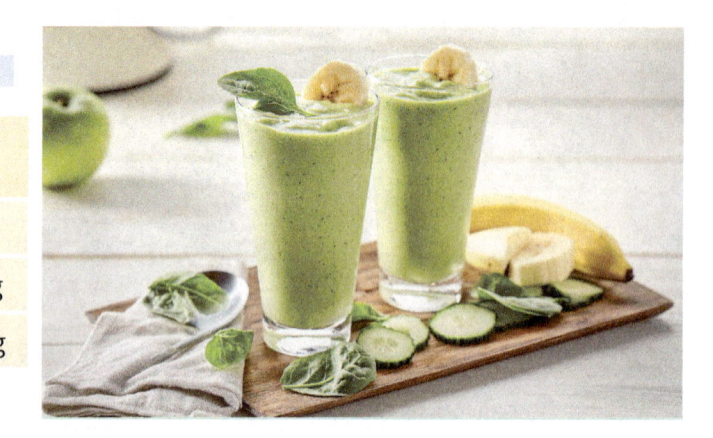

INGREDIENTS:
- 1 green apple (150 g)
- 1 small ripe banana (120 g)
- 1 cup fresh spinach (30 g)
- ½ cucumber (100 g)
- 1 tablespoon fresh lemon juice (15 ml)
- ¾ cup oat milk or unsweetened almond milk (180 ml)
- Ice cubes (optional)

INSTRUCTIONS:
1. Wash the spinach, apple, and cucumber. Core and chop the apple, peel and slice the cucumber, and peel the banana.
2. Add all the ingredients to a blender, including the lemon juice and plant-based milk.
3. Blend until smooth and silky.
4. Add a few ice cubes if you prefer it chilled, and blend again briefly.
5. Pour into tall glasses and serve immediately.
6. Optionally, garnish with a slice of cucumber or banana for a fresh touch.

BERRY YOGURT SHAKE WITH A TWIST

Servings: 2
Prep Time: 5 minutes
Cook Time: —

Nutrition Facts (per serving):
- Calories: 160
- Protein: 7 g
- Carbs: 25 g
- Fiber: 4 g
- Total Fat: 4 g
- Sodium: 75 mg

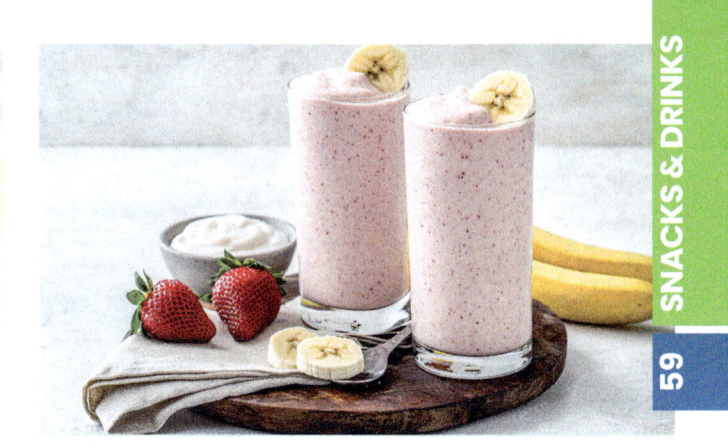

INGREDIENTS:
- 1 cup fresh strawberries, hulled (150 g)
- 1 ripe banana (120 g)
- 1 cup plain low-fat yogurt (240 g)
- ½ teaspoon vanilla extract (2 ml)
- 1/4 avocado (optional)
- Ice cubes (optional)

INSTRUCTIONS:
1. Peel the banana and slice the strawberries.
2. Add fruit, yogurt, vanilla, and avocado (if using) to a blender.
3. Blend until smooth and creamy.
4. Add ice if desired and blend again.
5. Serve immediately and enjoy.

EXPERT TIP:
Avocado adds creaminess and healthy fats—great for staying full and satisfied longer.

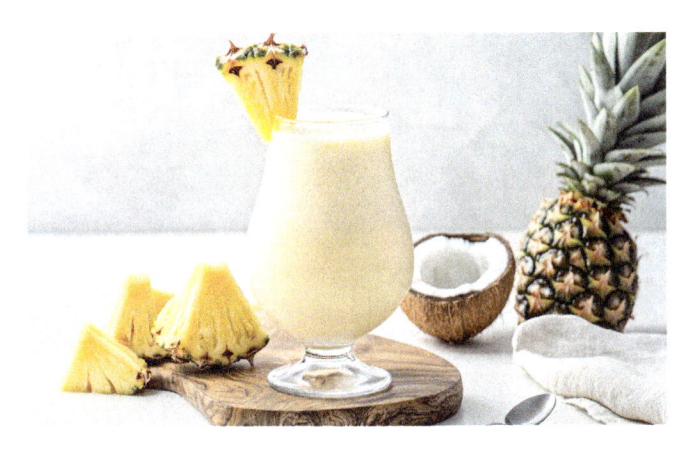

PIÑA COLADA DASH-FRIENDLY MOCKTAIL

Servings: 2
Prep Time: 5 minutes
Cook Time: —

Nutrition Facts (per serving):
- Calories: 120
- Protein: 4 g
- Carbs: 25 g
- Fiber: 3 g
- Total Fat: 2 g
- Sodium: 35 mg

INGREDIENTS:
- 1/2 cup fresh or frozen pineapple chunks (80 g)
- 1/2 cup coconut water (120 ml)
- 1/2 cup plain low-fat yogurt (120 g)
- 1/4 cup ice cubes (optional)
- 1 teaspoon vanilla extract (optional, for extra flavor)
- Pineapple slices or cherries for garnish (optional)

INSTRUCTIONS:
1. Add the pineapple, coconut water, yogurt, and ice (optional) to a blender.
2. Blend until smooth and creamy.
3. Taste and adjust the sweetness if necessary (you can add a bit of stevia if you want a sweeter taste).
4. Pour into two glasses, garnish with a slice of pineapple or a cherry, and serve immediately.

DID YOU KNOW?
Coconut water is rich in potassium and helps keep you hydrated—perfect for tropical drinks.

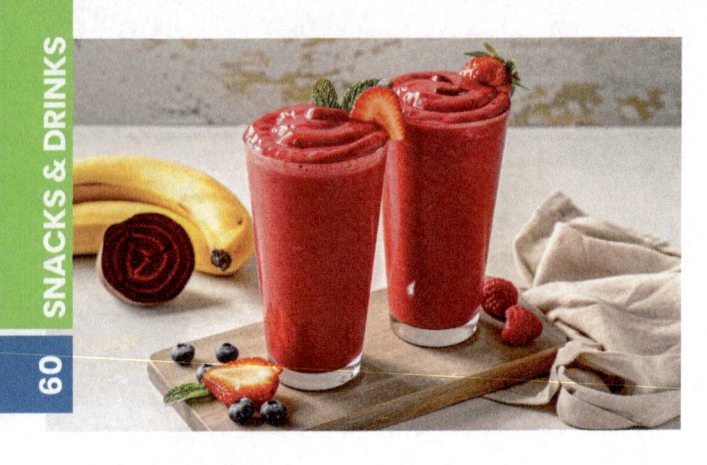

RED ANTIOXIDANT SMOOTHIE

Servings: 2

Prep Time: 5 minutes

Cook Time: —

Nutrition Facts (per serving):

Calories: 145	Fiber: 5 g
Protein: 3 g	Total Fat: 2 g
Carbs: 30 g	Sodium: 60 mg

INGREDIENTS:
- 1 small cooked beet (80 g)
- ¾ cup strawberries (fresh or frozen) (110 g)
- ½ cup raspberries or blueberries (75 g)
- 1 small ripe banana (120 g)
- ¾ cup oat milk or low-fat milk (180 ml)
- 1 tablespoon lemon juice (15 ml)
- Ice cubes (optional)

INSTRUCTIONS:
1. Peel and chop the cooked beet. Peel the banana. If using fresh berries, rinse them well.
2. Add the beet, strawberries, berries, banana, lemon juice, and milk to a blender.
3. Blend until smooth and creamy.
4. If needed, add a few ice cubes or more milk to adjust the consistency.
5. Pour into glasses and enjoy immediately.

DID YOU KNOW?
Beets are naturally rich in nitrates, which may help support healthy blood pressure—perfect for DASH!

PUMPKIN PIE SMOOTHIE

Servings: 2

Prep Time: 5 minutes

Cook Time: —

Nutrition Facts (per serving):

Calories: 130	Fiber: 4 g
Protein: 4 g	Total Fat: 3 g
Carbs: 22 g	Sodium: 60 mg

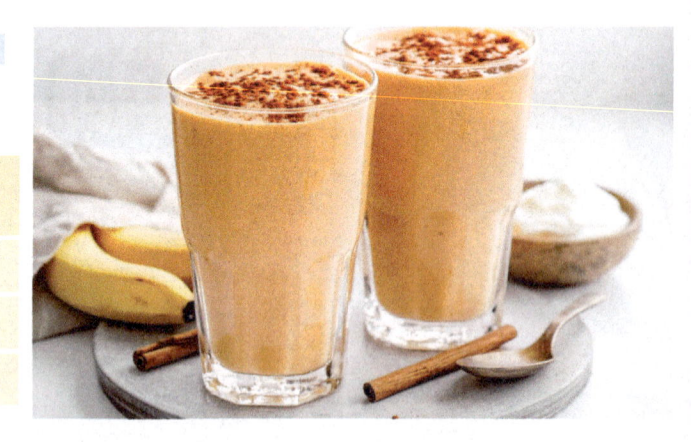

INGREDIENTS:
- ¾ cup canned pumpkin (unsweetened) (180 g)
- 1 small ripe banana (120 g)
- 1 cup unsweetened almond milk (240 ml)
- 2 tablespoons plain low-fat Greek yogurt (30 g)
- ½ teaspoon ground cinnamon (1 g)
- ¼ teaspoon ground nutmeg (0.5 g)
- ¼ teaspoon ground ginger (0.5 g)
- 1 teaspoon vanilla extract (5 ml)
- Ice cubes (optional)

INSTRUCTIONS:
1. Add the pumpkin, banana, almond milk, yogurt, spices, and vanilla to a blender.
2. Blend until completely smooth.
3. Add a few ice cubes if you prefer a colder texture and blend again.
4. Taste and adjust spices if needed.
5. Pour into two glasses and serve immediately. If desired, lightly dust with extra ground cinnamon on top for a festive touch!

EXPERT TIP
You can gently heat this smoothie (without boiling) for a cozy drink—like a spiced DASH-friendly latte.

DESSERTS

*Sweet treats made the DASH way—light, satisfying, and guilt-free.
End your meal with something sweet, simple, and heart-smart.*

DESSERTS

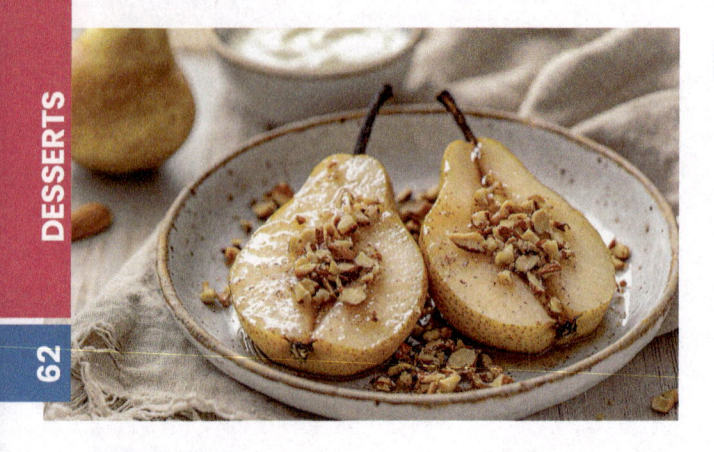

WARM CINNAMON-BAKED PEARS

Servings: 4

Prep Time: 10 minutes

Cook Time: 25 minutes

Nutrition Facts (per serving):

Calories: 165	Fiber: 4 g
Protein: 2 g	Total Fat: 7 g
Carbs: 24 g	Sodium: 3 mg

INGREDIENTS:

- 4 ripe pears (600 g)
- 2 tablespoons chopped almonds (20 g)
- 1 tablespoon olive oil (15 ml)
- 1 teaspoon ground cinnamon (2 g)
- 1 teaspoon vanilla extract (5 ml)
- 2 teaspoons maple syrup (optional)

INSTRUCTIONS:

1. Preheat the oven to 180°C (350°F).
2. Slice the pears in half and scoop out the cores with a spoon to create a small cavity.
3. In a small bowl, mix the chopped almonds, cinnamon, olive oil, and vanilla extract.
4. Spoon the mixture into the hollow of each pear half.
5. Place the pears in a baking dish and drizzle lightly with maple syrup, if desired.
6. Bake for 20–25 minutes, or until the pears are tender and the topping is golden.

ZESTY LEMON YOGURT MOUSSE

Servings: 4

Prep Time: 10 minutes

Cook Time: 2–3 hours

Nutrition Facts (per serving):

Calories: 155	Carbs: 24 g
Fat: 4 g	Fiber: 3 g
Sodium: 105 mg	Protein: 7 g

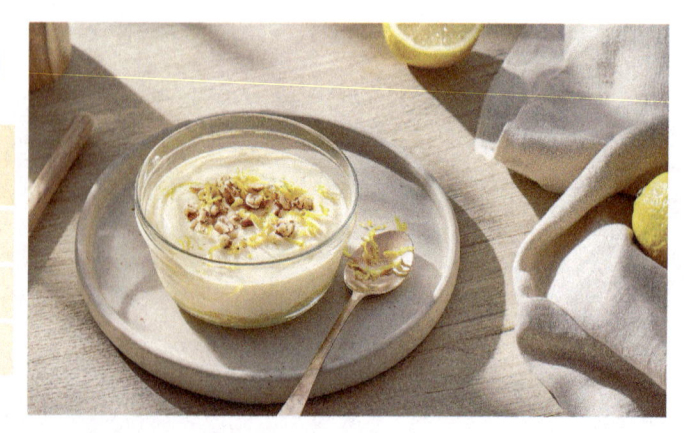

INGREDIENTS:

- ½ cup plain low-fat Greek yogurt (120 g)
- ¼ cup low-fat milk (60 ml)
- 1 tablespoon olive oil (optional, 15 ml)
- 2 tablespoons honey or maple syrup (30 ml)
- Juice of 1 lemon
- 1 teaspoon lemon zest
- ¾ cup whole wheat flour (75 g)
- 1 teaspoon baking powder (4 g)
- 1 egg
- ½ teaspoon vanilla extract
- Optional toppings: extra lemon zest or a few crushed unsalted nuts

INSTRUCTIONS:

1. Preheat the oven to 350°F (175°C).
2. In a mixing bowl, combine the flour and baking powder.
3. In another bowl, whisk the yogurt, milk, egg, honey, vanilla, lemon juice, and zest until smooth.
4. Add the wet ingredients to the dry and mix until just combined.
5. Pour into a small greased baking dish or divide the mixture between four small ramekins.
6. Bake for 20–25 minutes, or until set and slightly golden on top. Let cool before serving.

CHOCOLATE-DIPPED FRUIT SKEWERS

Servings: 4
Prep Time: 15 minutes
Cook Time: —

Nutrition Facts (per serving):
- Calories: 140
- Protein: 2 g
- Carbs: 20 g
- Fiber: 3 g
- Total Fat: 6 g
- Sodium: 5 mg

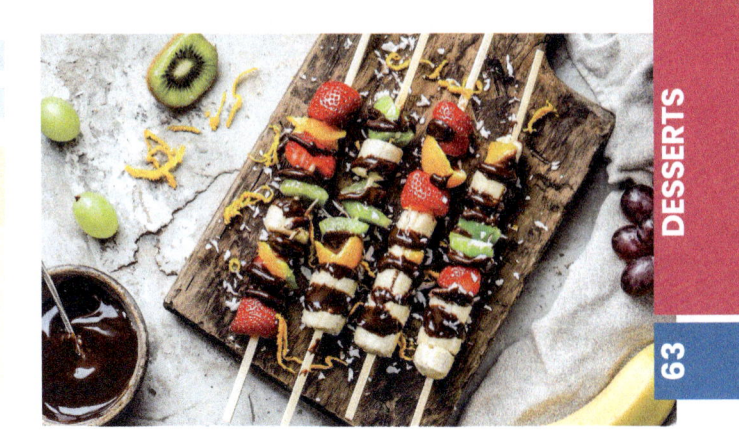

INGREDIENTS:
- 8–10 strawberries (100 g)
- 1 banana (120 g)
- 1 kiwi (75 g)
- 1 mandarin orange (80 g)
- 50 g dark chocolate (min. 70% cacao)
- 1 teaspoon orange zest or shredded coconut (optional)

INSTRUCTIONS:
1. Wash all the fruit. Peel the banana and kiwi.
2. Cut the fruit into bite-sized chunks and thread onto small wooden skewers.
3. Melt the dark chocolate in a microwave or over a bain-marie.
4. Drizzle the chocolate lightly over the skewers.
5. Sprinkle with orange zest or coconut if using.
6. Refrigerate for 10–15 minutes until the chocolate sets.

DASH TIP:
A sweet and colorful way to boost your fruit intake—perfect for guests or a quick treat!

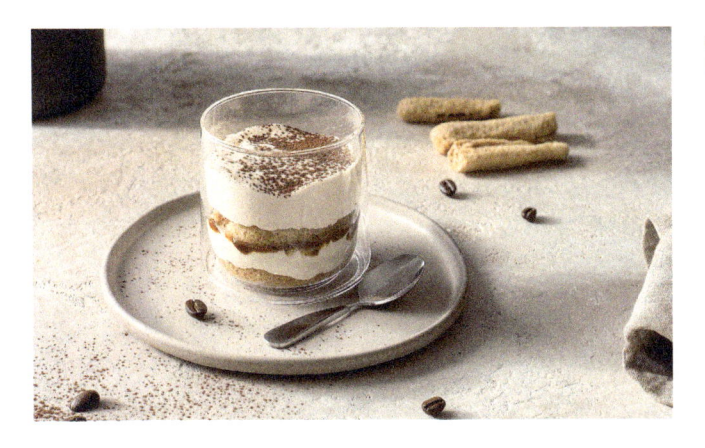

TIRAMISU IN A CUP

Servings: 4
Prep Time: 20 minutes
Cook Time: 2 hours

Nutrition Facts (per serving):
- Calories: 240
- Fat: 4g
- Sodium: 60mg
- Carbs: 40g
- Fiber: 7g
- Protein: 9g

INGREDIENTS:
- 12–14 light or low-sugar ladyfinger cookies (approx. 70 g)
- 1 cup plain Greek yogurt (low-fat) (240 g)
- ½ cup light ricotta cheese (120 g)
- 2 tablespoons maple syrup or honey (30 ml)
- 1 teaspoon vanilla extract (5 ml)
- ½ cup brewed coffee, cooled (120 ml)
- 1 tablespoon unsweetened cocoa powder (for dusting)

INSTRUCTIONS:
1. In a medium bowl, mix Greek yogurt, ricotta, maple syrup (or honey), and vanilla extract until smooth and creamy.
2. Dip each ladyfinger quickly into the cooled coffee (don't soak them—just a quick dip).
3. In 4 individual glasses, layer half the coffee-soaked ladyfingers on the bottom.
4. Spread half of the yogurt-ricotta cream over the ladyfingers.
5. Repeat the layers: remaining ladyfingers, then the rest of the cream.
6. Dust with cocoa powder. Cover and chill in the fridge for at least 2 hours before serving.

DASH TIP:
Can't find light ladyfingers? You can use thin slices of homemade whole-grain cake or low-sugar biscuits instead!

DESSERTS

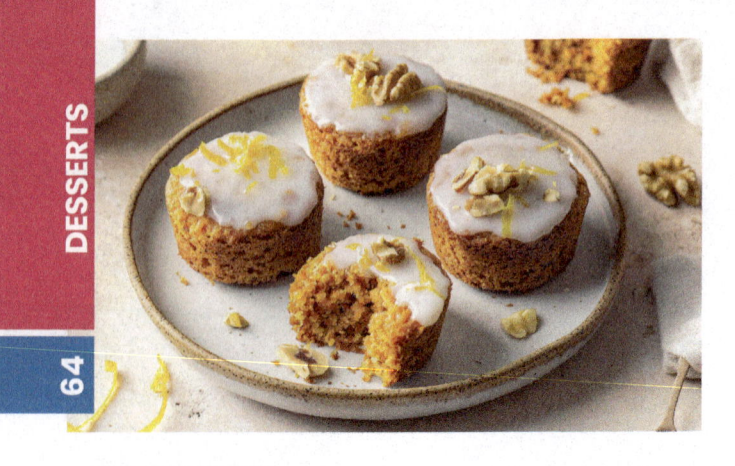

64

MINI CARROT & WALNUT CAKES

Servings: 4
Prep Time: 15 minutes
Cook Time: 25 minutes

Nutrition Facts (per serving):

Calories: 200	Fiber: 3 g
Protein: 5 g	Total Fat: 11 g
Carbs: 20 g	Sodium: 100 mg

INGREDIENTS:

- 1 cup grated carrot (90 g)
- 1 egg
- ⅓ cup whole wheat flour (40 g)
- ¼ cup chopped walnuts (20 g)
- 2 tablespoons raisins (20 g)
- 2 tablespoons olive oil (30 ml)
- 1 tablespoon maple syrup (15 ml)
- ½ teaspoon ground cinnamon (1 g)
- ½ teaspoon baking powder (2 g)

For the glaze:

- 2 tablespoons low-fat Greek yogurt (30 g)
- 1 teaspoon orange juice (5 ml)
- 1 teaspoon maple syrup (5 ml)
- Zest of ½ orange

INSTRUCTIONS:

1. Preheat oven to 175°C (350°F). Lightly grease 4 mini cake molds.
2. In a bowl, mix grated carrot, egg, olive oil, and maple syrup.
3. Add flour, cinnamon, baking powder, raisins, and walnuts. Stir to combine.
4. Divide the batter into the molds and bake for 20–25 minutes, until a toothpick comes out clean. Let cool completely.
5. In a small bowl, whisk the yogurt, orange juice, and maple syrup until smooth. Refrigerate for 10 minutes.
6. Let the cakes cool before topping with the glaze. Garnish with extra orange zest if desired.

CREAMY DASH CHEESECAKE

Servings: 4
Prep Time: 15 minutes
Cook Time: 25 minutes

Nutrition Facts (per serving):

Calories: 210	Carbs: 22 g
Fat: 8 g	Fiber: 2 g
Sodium: 90 mg	Protein: 12 g

INGREDIENTS:

For the crust:

- ½ cup whole wheat flour (60 g)
- 1 tablespoon olive oil (15 ml)
- 1 tablespoon honey or maple syrup (15 ml)
- 1 tablespoon milk or plant-based milk (15 ml)
- ½ teaspoon cinnamon

For the filling:

- 1 cup low-fat ricotta cheese (250 g)
- ½ cup low-fat plain Greek yogurt (120 g)
- 1 egg
- 1 tablespoon honey or maple syrup (15 ml)
- ½ teaspoon vanilla extract

INSTRUCTIONS:

1. Preheat oven to 175°C / 350°F.
2. In a bowl, combine whole wheat flour, olive oil, honey, milk, and cinnamon. Mix until a dough forms.
3. Press the dough evenly into the bottom of a small baking dish (or four ramekins). Bake for 8–10 minutes, then remove and let it cool slightly.
4. Meanwhile, prepare the filling: blend ricotta, yogurt, egg, honey, and vanilla until smooth.
5. Pour the filling over the crust and bake for 15–18 minutes, until set but still slightly wobbly in the center.
6. Let cool completely, then refrigerate for at least 2–3 hours. Add toppings just before serving (strawberries, blueberries, mango, kiwi, or other fresh fruit).

CHOCOLATE PISTACHIO OAT COOKIES

Servings: 12

Prep Time: 10 minutes

Cook Time: 15 minutes

Nutrition Facts (per serving):

Calories: 85 | Carbs: 10g
Fat: 4g | Fiber: 1.5g
Sodium: 40mg | Protein: 2g

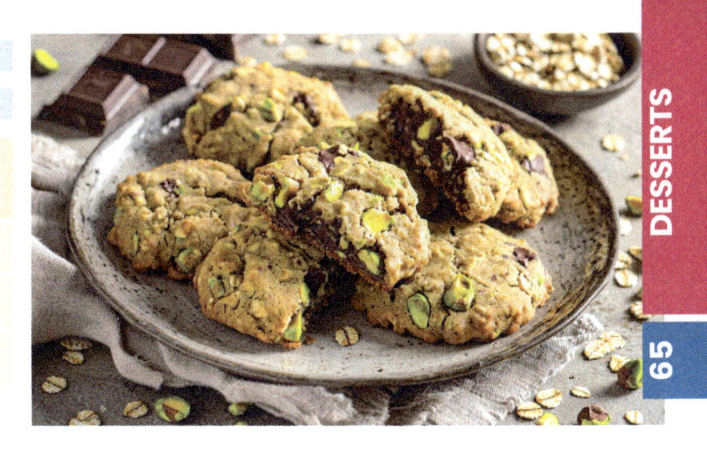

INGREDIENTS:

- 1 cup rolled oats (90 g)
- ⅓ cup almond flour (35 g)
- ¼ teaspoon ground cinnamon (0.5 g)
- ½ teaspoon baking powder (2 g)
- 1 ripe banana, mashed (120 g)
- 1 tablespoon maple syrup or honey (15 ml)
- 1 teaspoon vanilla extract (5 ml)
- 2 tablespoons pistachios (20 g)
- 2 tablespoons dark chocolate (min. 70%, no added sugar) (20 g)

INSTRUCTIONS:

1. Preheat the oven to 350°F (175°C) and line a baking sheet with parchment paper.
2. In a large bowl, mix the oats, almond flour, cinnamon, and baking powder.
3. In a separate bowl, combine the mashed banana, maple syrup, and vanilla extract.
4. Add the wet mixture to the dry ingredients and stir until fully combined.
5. Fold in the chopped pistachios and dark chocolate.
6. Scoop out portions of the dough and shape into small cookies. Place them on the baking sheet and flatten slightly. Bake for 12–15 minutes or until lightly golden. Let cool before serving.

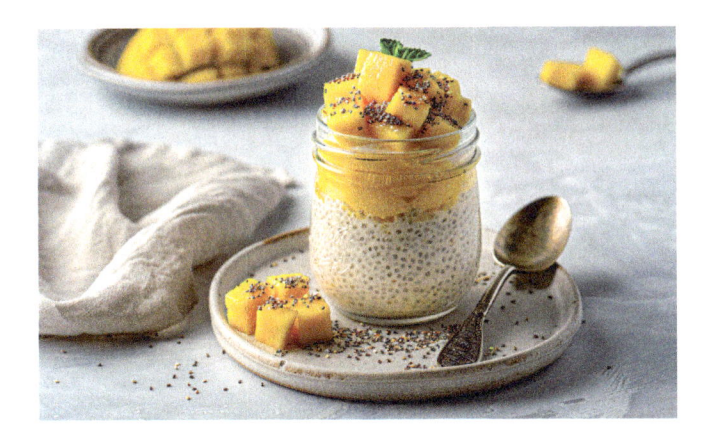

CHIA & MANGO PUDDING

Servings: 4

Prep Time: 5 minutes

Cook Time: 4 hours

Nutrition Facts (per serving):

Calories: 160 | Fiber: 8 g
Protein: 4 g | Total Fat: 7 g
Carbs: 20 g | Sodium: 80 mg

INGREDIENTS:

- 6 tablespoons chia seeds (60 g)
- 2 cups unsweetened almond milk or oat milk (480 ml)
- 2 teaspoons honey or maple syrup (14 g), optional
- 1 teaspoon vanilla extract (5 ml)
- 1 cup ripe mango, mashed with a fork (200 g)

INSTRUCTIONS:

1. In a medium bowl or jar, combine chia seeds, plant-based milk, vanilla, and sweetener if using.
2. Stir well to prevent clumping. Let sit for 5 minutes, then stir again.
3. Cover and refrigerate for at least 4 hours or overnight, until thickened.
4. Before serving, stir again and divide into four bowls or glasses.
5. Top with the mashed mango and enjoy cold.

DID YOU KNOW?

Chia seeds absorb up to 10 times their weight in liquid, turning into a natural thickener—no need for gelatin!

DESSERTS

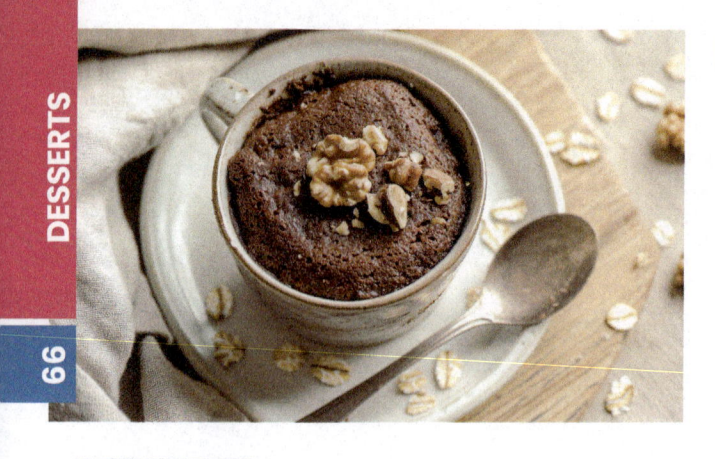

66

COCOA & WALNUT MUG CAKE

Servings: 4
Prep Time: 5 minutes
Cook Time: 2 minutes

Nutrition Facts (per serving):

Calories: 160	Carbs: 19g
Fat: 8g	Fiber: 3g
Sodium: 100mg	Protein: 5g

INGREDIENTS:
- 2 eggs
- 6 tablespoons unsweetened oat milk (90 ml)
- 6 tablespoons unsweetened applesauce (90 g)
- 6 tablespoons whole wheat flour (50 g)
- 4 teaspoons unsweetened cocoa powder (10 g)
- 1 teaspoon baking powder
- ½ teaspoon ground cinnamon
- 4 tablespoons walnuts (40 g)

INSTRUCTIONS:
1. In a mixing bowl, whisk the eggs with oat milk and applesauce.
2. Stir in flour, cocoa powder, baking powder, and cinnamon. Mix until smooth.
3. Fold in the chopped walnuts.
4. Divide the mixture into four microwave-safe mugs.
5. Microwave each mug (one at a time) on high for 1½ to 2 minutes, or until the center is just set.
6. Let cool slightly and enjoy warm.

EXPERT TIP:
Sweetened only with applesauce, this cozy treat is DASH-friendly and ready in just minutes.

RHUBARB & PECAN MUFFINS

Servings: 6 muffins
Prep Time: 10 minutes
Cook Time: 20 minutes

Nutrition Facts (per serving):

Calories: 170	Carbs: 17g
Fat: 9g	Fiber: 2g
Sodium: 115mg	Protein: 4g

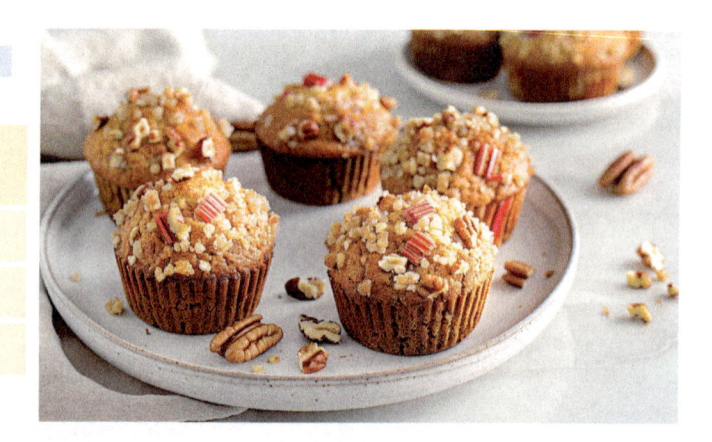

INGREDIENTS:
- 1 egg
- ½ cup low-fat plain yogurt (125 g)
- ¼ cup light olive oil (60 ml)
- ¼ cup brown sugar (30 g)
- 1 teaspoon vanilla extract
- ¾ cup whole wheat flour (75 g)
- ½ teaspoon baking soda
- ½ teaspoon ground cinnamon
- ¾ cup rhubarb (90 g)
- 2 tablespoons pecans (15 g)

INSTRUCTIONS:
1. Preheat the oven to 350°F (180°C). Line or lightly grease a muffin tin with 6 molds.
2. In a bowl, whisk the egg with yogurt, oil, sugar, and vanilla until smooth.
3. Add flour, baking soda, and cinnamon. Stir until just combined.
4. Gently fold in the rhubarb and chopped pecans.
5. Divide the batter evenly into the muffin molds.
6. Bake for 18–20 minutes or until a toothpick inserted into the center comes out clean. Let cool on a wire rack before serving.

AMERICAN-STYLE APPLE CRUMBLE

Servings: 4
Prep Time: 10 minutes
Cook Time: 30 minutes

Nutrition Facts (per serving):
Calories: 210 Carbs: 28g
Fat: 10g Fiber: 4g
Sodium: 35mg Protein: 3g

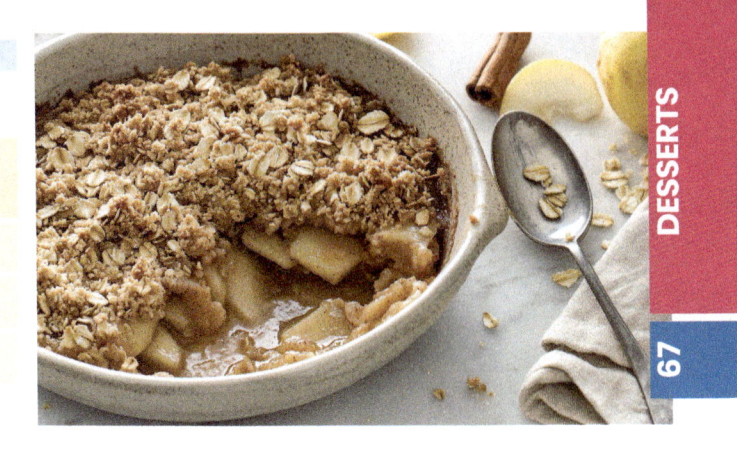

INGREDIENTS:

- 3 medium apples, peeled and sliced (approx. 360 g)
- 1 tablespoon lemon juice (15 ml)
- ½ teaspoon ground cinnamon (1 g)
- ½ cup rolled oats (40 g)
- 2 tablespoons whole wheat flour (16 g)
- 2 tablespoons olive oil (30 ml)
- 2 tablespoons chopped walnuts or pecans (15 g)
- 1 teaspoon maple syrup (5 ml) (optional)

INSTRUCTIONS:

1. Preheat the oven to 180°C (350°F).
2. In a bowl, toss the sliced apples with lemon juice and cinnamon.
3. Spread the apples evenly in a small baking dish.
4. In another bowl, mix oats, flour, olive oil, and nuts until crumbly. Add maple syrup if desired.
5. Sprinkle the crumble topping over the apples.
6. Bake for about 30 minutes, or until the apples are tender and the topping is golden and crisp.

DASH TIP:

This classic dessert skips added sugar in the filling—let the natural sweetness of apples shine!

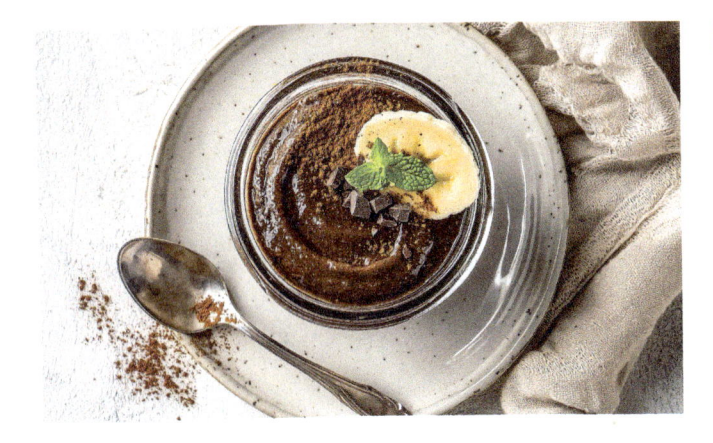

LIGHT CHOCOLATE PUDDING

Servings: 4
Prep Time: 10 minutes
Cook Time: None

Nutrition Facts (per serving):
Calories: 240 Carbs: 40g
Fat: 4g Fiber: 7g
Sodium: 60mg Protein: 9g

INGREDIENTS:

- 1 ripe avocado (150 g)
- 1 medium ripe banana (120 g)
- 2 tablespoons unsweetened cocoa powder (16 g)
- 3 tablespoons plain low-fat yogurt (45 g)
- 1 teaspoon vanilla extract (5 ml)

INSTRUCTIONS:

1. Peel the banana and avocado, then add them to a food processor.
2. Add the cocoa powder, yogurt, and vanilla extract.
3. Blend until completely smooth and creamy.
4. Taste and adjust sweetness with a touch of mashed banana if needed.
5. Spoon into small serving glasses or ramekins.
6. Chill for at least 1 hour before serving. Top with a banana slice or a pinch of cocoa powder before serving, if desired.

DASH TIP:

This pudding has a creamy, mousse-like texture thanks to the avocado—no need for added sugar or cream!

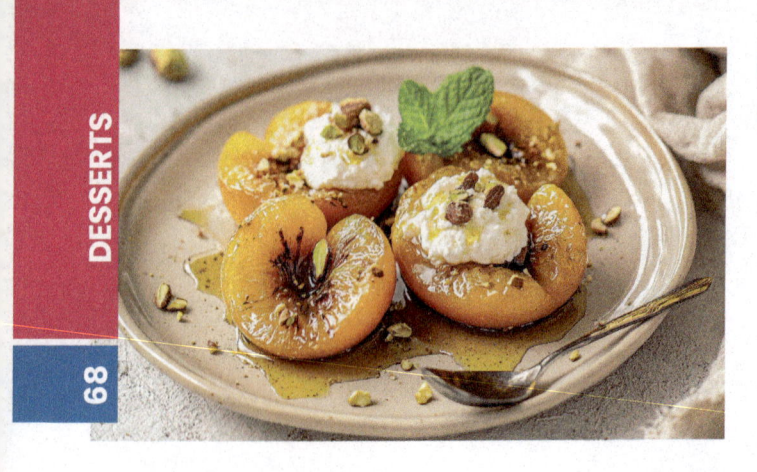

MEDITERRANEAN BAKED APRICOTS WITH A TWIST

Servings: 4
Prep Time: 5 minutes
Cook Time: 15 minutes

Nutrition Facts (per serving):

Calories: 120	Carbs: 16g
Fat: 4g	Fiber: 2g
Sodium: 55mg	Protein: 5g

INGREDIENTS:

- 8 fresh apricots
- 1 teaspoon olive oil (5 ml)
- 1 teaspoon ground cinnamon
- ⅔ cup light ricotta cheese (160 g)
- 2 teaspoons honey (14 g)
- Optional: pistachios or fresh mint for garnish

INSTRUCTIONS:

1. Preheat the oven to 180°C (350°F).
2. Arrange the apricot halves in a baking dish, cut side up.
3. Lightly brush the apricots with olive oil and sprinkle with cinnamon.
4. Bake for 12–15 minutes until tender and slightly caramelized.
5. Remove from the oven and let cool for a few minutes.
6. Serve warm with a dollop of ricotta on each half and a drizzle of honey. Garnish with crushed pistachios or mint if desired.

EXPERT TIP:

No apricots? Try peaches instead—they bake just as well and match the Mediterranean vibe perfectly.

WARM BERRY CRISP WITH OAT TOPPING

Servings: 4
Prep Time: 10 minutes
Cook Time: 25 minutes

Nutrition Facts (per serving):

Calories: 195	Fiber: 4 g
Protein: 3 g	Total Fat: 9 g
Carbs: 25 g	Sodium: 25 mg

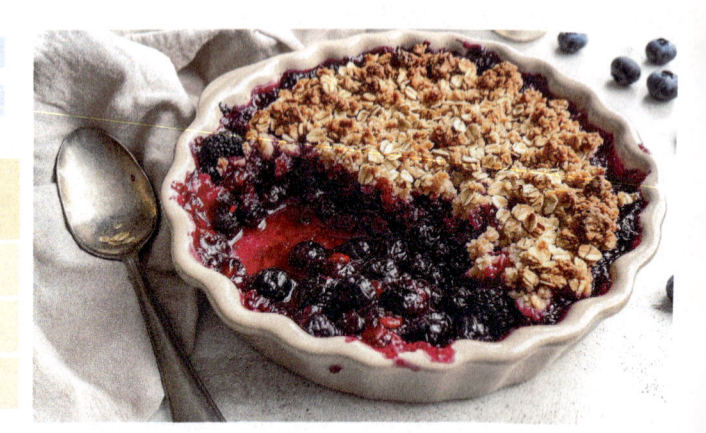

INGREDIENTS:

- 2 cups mixed berries (fresh or frozen, 280 g) – e.g. blueberries, raspberries, blackberries
- 1 teaspoon lemon juice (5 ml)
- ½ cup rolled oats (40 g)
- 2 tablespoons whole wheat flour (16 g)
- 2 tablespoons olive oil (30 ml)
- 1 tablespoon almonds (8 g)
- 1 teaspoon honey or maple syrup (optional, 5 ml)

INSTRUCTIONS:

1. Preheat the oven to 180°C (350°F).
2. In a small baking dish, mix the berries with the lemon juice and spread them evenly.
3. In a bowl, combine oats, flour, olive oil, chopped almonds, and honey or maple syrup if using. Mix until crumbly.
4. Sprinkle the crumble mixture over the berries.
5. Bake for 25 minutes, or until the topping is golden and the berries are bubbly.
6. Let cool slightly before serving. Serve warm or at room temperature.

DID YOU KNOW?

Mixed berries add natural color and sweetness—plus antioxidants that support heart and brain health.

MEDITERRANEAN EGGPLANT DIP (BABA GANOUSH)

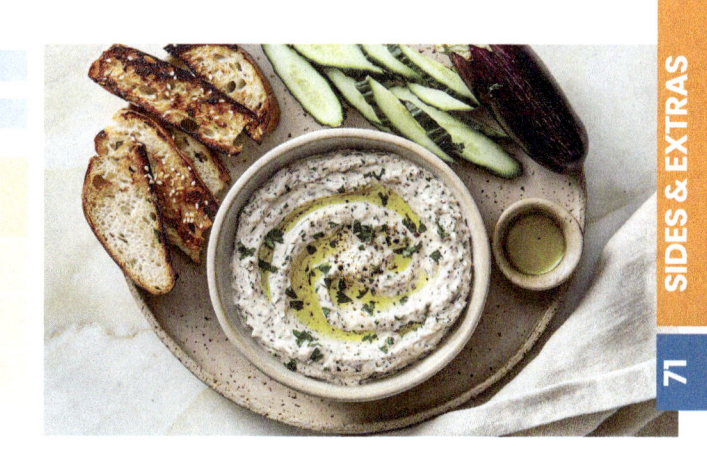

Servings: 4
Prep Time: 10 minutes
Cook Time: 35 minutes

Nutrition Facts (per serving):
- Calories: 110
- Fat: 7g
- Sodium: 20mg
- Carbs: 11g
- Fiber: 5g
- Protein: 3g

INGREDIENTS:
- 2 medium eggplants (approx. 18 oz / 500 g)
- 2 tablespoons tahini (30 g)
- 1 tablespoon fresh lemon juice (15 ml)
- 1 small garlic clove, minced
- 1 tablespoon extra-virgin olive oil (15 ml)
- Black pepper to taste
- Fresh parsley, chopped (optional)

INSTRUCTIONS:
1. Preheat the oven to 400°F (200°C). Cut the eggplants in half lengthwise and place them cut-side down on a baking sheet lined with parchment paper.
2. Bake for 30–35 minutes, or until very tender. Let cool slightly.
3. Scoop out the eggplant flesh with a spoon and place it into a bowl.
4. Add tahini, lemon juice, garlic, and olive oil. Mash well with a fork or briefly process until smooth and creamy.
5. Season with pepper to taste. Garnish with chopped parsley if desired.
6. Serve at room temperature or chilled, paired with toasted whole-grain bread or fresh veggie sticks.

DID YOU KNOW?
Baba Ganoush is a Mediterranean classic rich in fiber and antioxidants—perfect for your heart!

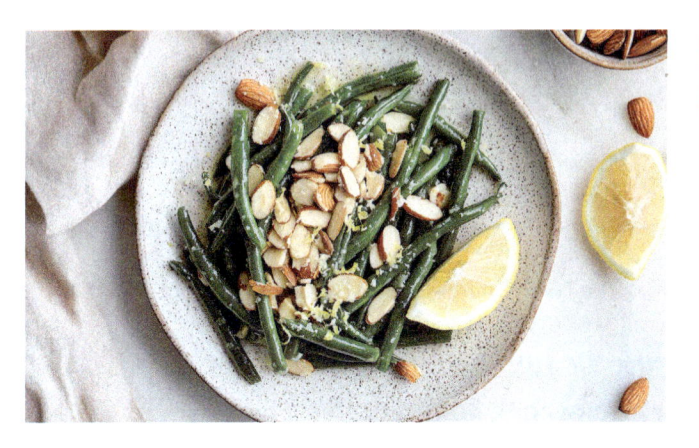

GREEN BEANS WITH TOASTED ALMONDS

Servings: 4
Prep Time: 10 minutes
Cook Time: 8 minutes

Nutrition Facts (per serving):
- Calories: 240
- Fat: 4g
- Sodium: 60mg
- Carbs: 40g
- Fiber: 7g
- Protein: 9g

INGREDIENTS:
- 300 g green beans
- 2 tablespoons unsalted almonds (15 g)
- 1 tablespoon olive oil (15 ml)
- Juice of ½ lemon
- Zest of ½ lemon
- Black pepper to taste

INSTRUCTIONS:
1. Steam or boil the green beans for 5–6 minutes until just tender and bright green. Drain well.
2. In a large skillet, toast the almonds over medium heat for 2–3 minutes until golden. Transfer to a plate and set aside.
3. In the same skillet, heat the olive oil. Add the green beans and sauté for 1–2 minutes.
4. Add the lemon juice, zest, and black pepper. Toss gently to combine.
5. Top with the toasted almonds and serve warm or at room temperature.

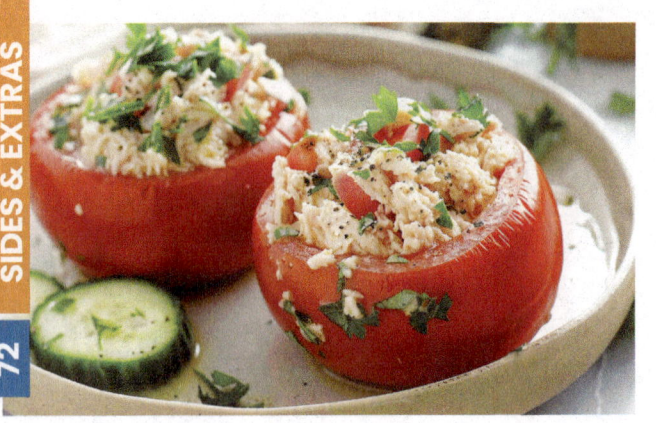

MEDITERRANEAN TOMATO & TUNA BITES

Servings: 4
Prep Time: 10 minutes
Cook Time: —

Nutrition Facts (per serving):

Calories: 160	Carbs: 4g
Fat: 8g	Fiber: 1g
Sodium: 130mg	Protein: 18g

INGREDIENTS:
- 4 small ripe tomatoes (400 g)
- 2 hard-boiled eggs (100 g)
- 2 cans low-sodium tuna in water, drained (8 oz / 240 g)
- 2 teaspoons olive oil (10 ml)
- 2 tablespoons parsley (optional)
- Black pepper to taste

INSTRUCTIONS:
1. Boil the eggs in advance and let them cool.
2. Slice the tops off the tomatoes and gently scoop out the inside with a small spoon.
3. In a bowl, mash the hard-boiled eggs with the drained tuna and olive oil. Add black pepper to taste and mix until creamy.
4. Fill each tomato with the tuna mixture using a small spoon.
5. Sprinkle with chopped parsley if desired, and serve chilled.

SERVING TIP:
Use ripe, firm tomatoes to avoid sogginess. You can also serve the mix over cucumber slices for extra crunch.

ROASTED BUTTERNUT SQUASH WITH A TWIST

Servings: 4
Prep Time: 15 minutes
Cook Time: 30 minutes

Nutrition Facts (per serving):

Calories: 220	Carbs: 30g
Fat: 9g	Fiber: 5g
Sodium: 40mg	Protein: 5g

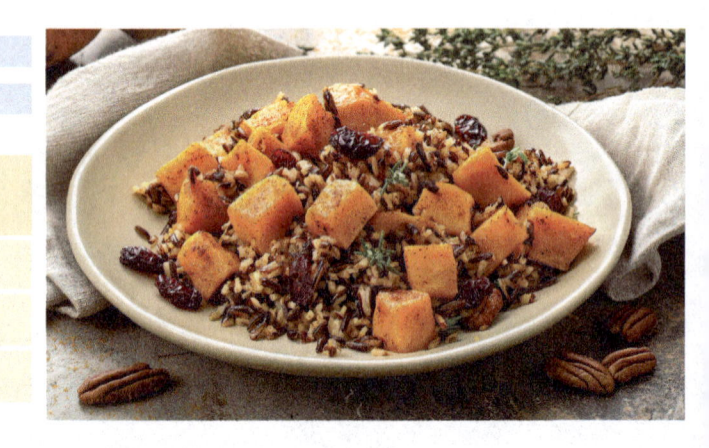

INGREDIENTS:
- 2 cups cubed butternut squash (300 g)
- 1 tablespoon olive oil (15 ml)
- 1 cup cooked wild rice (160 g)
- 1 cup cooked brown rice (160 g)
- 2 tablespoons dried cranberries (20 g)
- 2 tablespoons unsalted pecans (15 g)
- ½ teaspoon dried thyme (1 g)
- ¼ teaspoon ground cinnamon
- Black pepper to taste

INSTRUCTIONS:
1. Preheat oven to 400°F (200°C).
2. Toss the cubed butternut squash with olive oil, thyme, cinnamon, and black pepper. Spread on a baking sheet.
3. Roast for 25–30 minutes, or until tender and lightly golden.
4. In a large bowl, combine the roasted squash with the wild rice, brown rice, cranberries, and chopped pecans.
5. Mix gently to combine and serve warm.

SERVING TIP:
This side dish pairs perfectly with roast turkey or baked salmon and makes a great addition to holiday meals.

SAUTÉED KALE WITH CHERRY TOMATOES

Servings: 4
Prep Time: 10 minutes
Cook Time: 10 minutes

Nutrition Facts (per serving):

Calories: 90	Carbs: 8g
Fat: 6g	Fiber: 3g
Sodium: 40mg	Protein: 3g

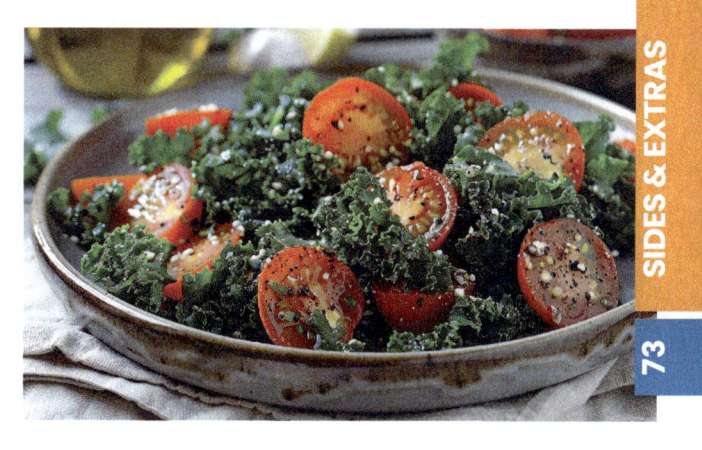

INGREDIENTS:

- 1 tablespoon olive oil (15 ml)
- 1 garlic clove (3 g)
- 4 cups chopped kale, stems removed (100 g)
- 1 cup halved cherry tomatoes (150 g)
- Juice of ½ lemon
- Black pepper to taste
- 1 teaspoon white sesame seeds (3 g), optional

INSTRUCTIONS:

1. Mince the garlic.
2. Heat olive oil in a large skillet over medium heat. Add the garlic and cook for 1 minute.
3. Add the chopped kale and sauté for about 4–5 minutes, stirring frequently, until wilted.
4. Stir in the cherry tomatoes and cook for another 3–4 minutes, until softened.
5. Finish with lemon juice and a touch of black pepper and sprinkle with sesame seeds before serving, if desired.
6. Serve warm and enjoy!

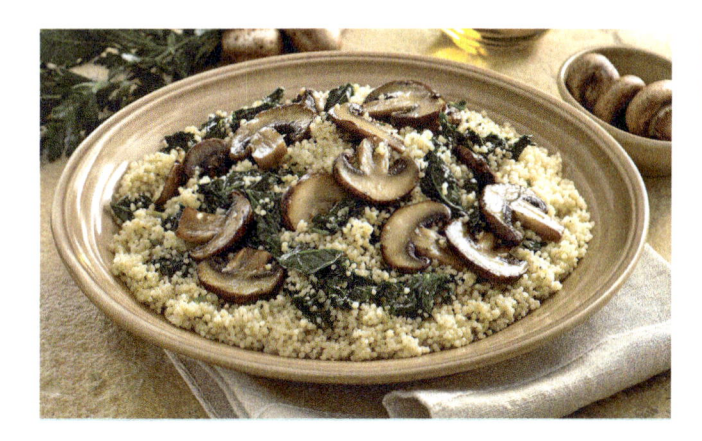

NOURISHING COUSCOUS WITH MUSHROOMS & SWISS CHARD

Servings: 4
Prep Time: 10 minutes
Cook Time: 25 minutes

Nutrition Facts (per serving):

Calories: 190	Carbs: 30g
Fat: 6g	Fiber: 5g
Sodium: 140mg	Protein: 6g

INGREDIENTS:

- 1 tablespoon olive oil (15 ml)
- 1 small onion (80 g)
- 1 garlic clove (3 g)
- 1 cup couscous (180 g)
- 2 cups low-sodium vegetable broth (475 ml)
- 1 cup mushrooms (100 g)
- 1 cup Swiss chard (200 g)
- Black pepper to taste

INSTRUCTIONS:

1. Peel and finely chop the onion and garlic. Slice the mushrooms and chop the Swiss chard.
2. In a saucepan, heat olive oil over medium heat. Sauté onion and garlic for 2–3 minutes, until fragrant.
3. Add the mushrooms and cook for another 4–5 minutes, until they begin to soften.
4. Stir in the couscous and toast for 1–2 minutes, stirring often.
5. Pour in the vegetable broth and bring to a boil. Reduce heat, cover, and simmer for about 5–7 minutes, or until the couscous absorbs the liquid.
6. Add the Swiss chard in the last 2 minutes of cooking, allowing it to soften and mix in with the couscous.
7. Fluff with a fork, season with pepper, and fold in the fresh herbs just before serving.

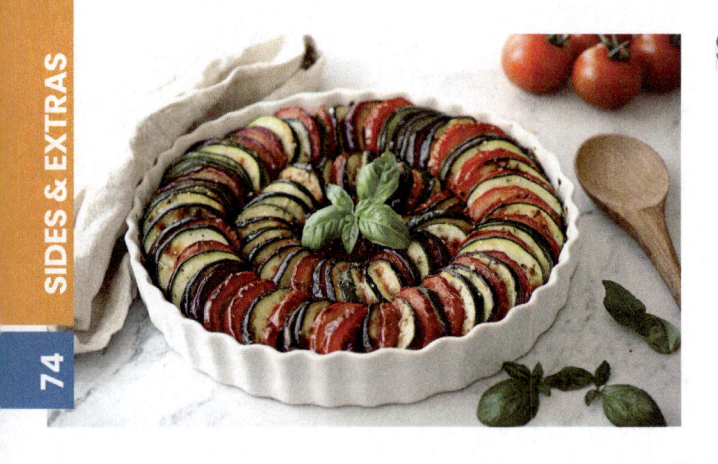

SIMPLE RATATOUILLE BAKE

Servings: 4
Prep Time: 15 minutes
Cook Time: 35 minutes

Nutrition Facts (per serving):

Calories: 115	Carbs: 12g
Fat: 7g	Fiber: 4g
Sodium: 85mg	Protein: 2g

INGREDIENTS:
- 1 small eggplant (200 g)
- 1 zucchini (150 g)
- 1 red bell pepper (120 g)
- 2 ripe tomatoes (250 g total)
- 1 cup low-sodium crushed tomatoes (240 g)
- 1 garlic clove, minced (3 g)
- 2 tablespoons extra virgin olive oil (30 ml)
- 1 teaspoon dried thyme (1 g)
- 1 teaspoon dried oregano (1 g)
- Black pepper to taste

INSTRUCTIONS:
1. Preheat the oven to 190°C (375°F).
2. Peel and mince the garlic. Thinly slice the eggplant, zucchini, tomatoes, and bell pepper into even rounds.
3. Spread the crushed tomatoes in the bottom of a baking dish. Add the minced garlic and half of the herbs. Stir gently to combine.
4. Arrange the vegetable slices over the sauce in alternating layers (eggplant, zucchini, tomato, bell pepper), slightly overlapping in a spiral or straight rows.
5. Drizzle with olive oil and sprinkle with the remaining herbs and black pepper.
6. Cover loosely with foil and bake for 25 minutes. Uncover and bake for another 10 minutes until the vegetables are tender and slightly golden. Garnish with fresh basil if desired.

BASIL-GINGER STUFFED MUSHROOMS

Servings: 4
Prep Time: 15 minutes
Cook Time: 20 minutes

Nutrition Facts (per serving):

Calories: 110	Carbs: 6g
Fat: 8g	Fiber: 2g
Sodium: 75mg	Protein: 4g

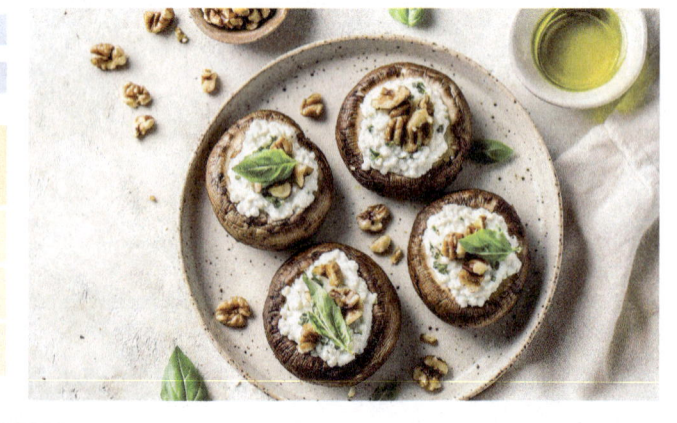

INGREDIENTS:
- 12 medium cremini or white mushrooms (300 g)
- 2 tablespoons extra virgin olive oil (30 ml)
- 1 small garlic clove (3 g)
- 1 teaspoon fresh ginger (5 g)
- 2 tablespoons fresh basil (5 g)
- 1 tablespoon walnuts (7 g)
- 2 tablespoons low-sodium cottage cheese (30 g)
- 1 tablespoon lemon juice (15 ml)
- Black pepper to taste

INSTRUCTIONS:
1. Preheat the oven to 190°C (375°F). Clean the mushrooms with a damp cloth, remove the stems, and finely chop them.
2. Mince the garlic and grate the ginger. Chop the basil.
3. Heat 1 tablespoon olive oil in a pan over medium heat. Sauté the chopped stems, garlic, and ginger for 5–6 minutes until soft.
4. Remove from heat. Stir in basil, walnuts, cottage cheese, lemon juice, and pepper. Mix well.
5. Fill each mushroom cap with the mixture and place on a lined tray.
6. Drizzle with remaining oil and bake for 15 minutes, or until tender and lightly golden.

ROASTED CARROT & PARSNIP WEDGES WITH THYME

Servings: 4
Prep Time: 10 minutes
Cook Time: 25 minutes

Nutrition Facts (per serving):
- Calories: 130
- Protein: 4 g
- Carbs: 10 g
- Fiber: 4 g
- Total Fat: 9 g
- Sodium: 20 mg

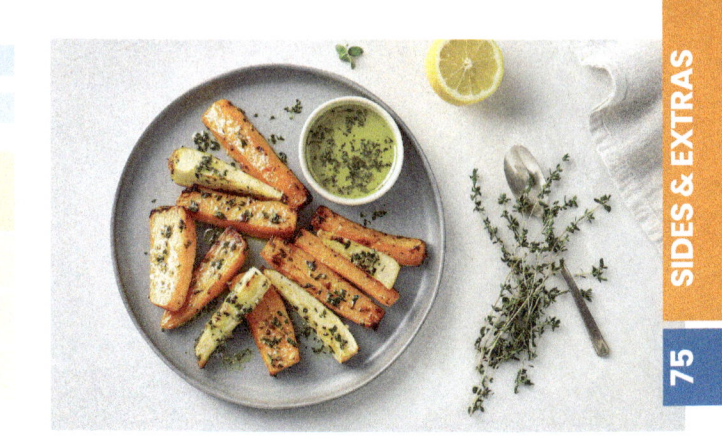

INGREDIENTS:
- 3 medium carrots (300 g)
- 2 medium parsnips (300 g)
- 1 tablespoon olive oil (15 ml)
- 1 teaspoon fresh thyme or ½ teaspoon dried thyme
- ¼ teaspoon black pepper (0.5 g)
- For the Lemon-Herb Dressing:
- 2 tablespoons lemon juice (30 ml)
- 1 teaspoon Dijon mustard (5 ml)
- 2 tablespoons olive oil (30 ml)
- 1 teaspoon chopped parsley or thyme
- Black pepper to taste

INSTRUCTIONS:
1. Preheat the oven to 200°C (400°F).
2. Peel the carrots and parsnips, then cut them into thick wedges.
3. Toss the wedges with olive oil, thyme, and pepper. Spread them evenly on a baking tray.
4. Roast for 25 minutes, flipping halfway through, until golden and tender.
5. Meanwhile, mix all the dressing ingredients in a small jar and shake well.
6. Drizzle the dressing over the roasted veggies just before serving or serve it on the side.

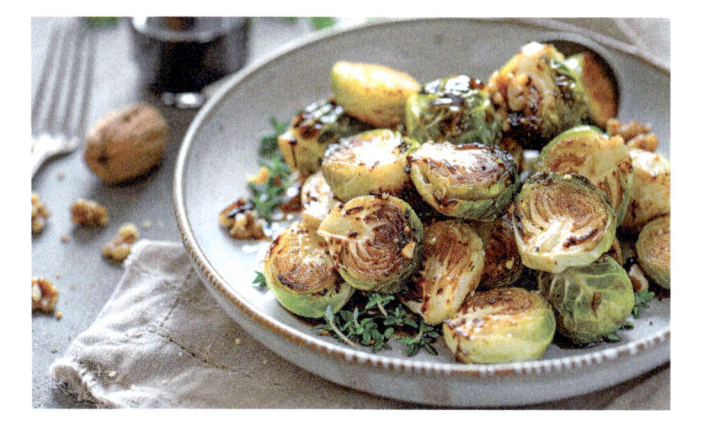

BALSAMIC ROASTED BRUSSELS SPROUTS WITH WALNUTS

Servings: 4
Prep Time: 10 minutes
Cook Time: 25 minutes

Nutrition Facts (per serving):
- Calories: 240
- Fat: 4g
- Sodium: 60mg
- Carbs: 40g
- Fiber: 7g
- Protein: 9g

INGREDIENTS:
- 450 g Brussels sprouts
- 1 tablespoon olive oil (15 ml)
- Black pepper to taste
- 1 tablespoon balsamic vinegar (15 ml)
- 2 tablespoons walnuts (15 g)

INSTRUCTIONS:
1. Preheat the oven to 200°C (400°F).
2. Trim the Brussels sprouts and cut them in half.
3. Toss them with olive oil and black pepper until evenly coated.
4. Spread on a parchment-lined baking sheet and roast for 20–25 minutes, stirring once halfway through.
5. Remove from the oven and immediately drizzle with the balsamic vinegar while still hot.
6. Sprinkle with walnuts and serve warm.

DID YOU KNOW?

Brussels sprouts and walnuts are a fiber-rich combo that supports heart health and helps stabilize blood sugar.

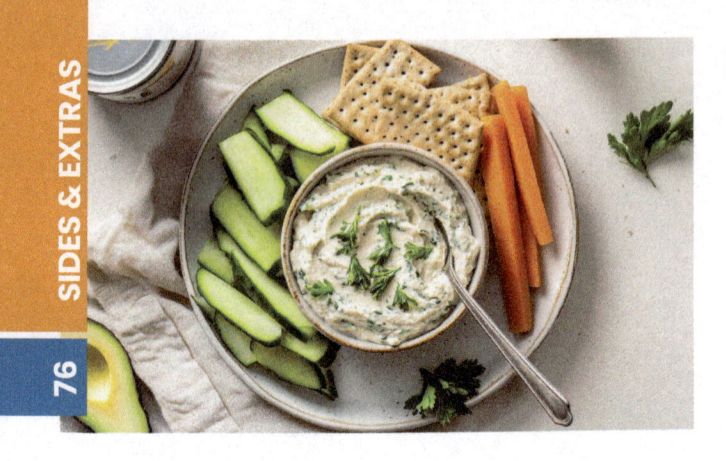

CREAMY TUNA SPREAD

Servings: 4
Prep Time: 8 minutes
Cook Time: —

Nutrition Facts (per serving):

Calories: 110	Fiber: 1 g
Protein: 12 g	Total Fat: 5 g
Carbs: 2 g	Sodium: 100 mg

INGREDIENTS:

- 1 can no-salt-added tuna (approx. 140 g)
- 2 tablespoons plain low-fat yogurt (30 g)
- ¼ ripe avocado (30 g)
- 1 teaspoon lemon juice (5 ml)
- 1 tablespoon finely chopped celery (10 g)
- 1 tablespoon chopped fresh parsley (optional)
- Black pepper to taste

INSTRUCTIONS:

1. Drain the tuna and place it in a medium bowl.
2. Add the yogurt, avocado, and lemon juice.
3. Mash everything together with a fork until creamy but still slightly chunky.
4. Stir in the celery, parsley (if using), and black pepper.
5. Adjust the texture or seasoning if needed.
6. Serve chilled with whole grain crackers or veggie sticks.

SERVING TIP:
This spread combines protein and healthy fats, making it perfect as a dip or sandwich filling.

PICKLED ONION & CARROT SLAW

Servings: 4
Prep Time: 10 minutes
Cook Time: 30 min. (or overnight for stronger flavor)

Nutrition Facts (per serving):

Calories: 35	Fiber: 1 g
Protein: 0 g	Total Fat: 0 g
Carbs: 8 g	Sodium: 15 mg

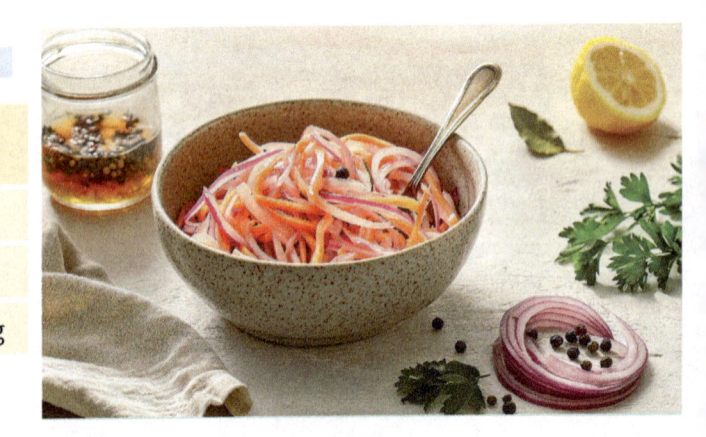

INGREDIENTS:

- 1 small red onion (80 g)
- 1 large carrot (100 g)
- ½ cup white or apple cider vinegar (120 ml)
- ¼ cup water (60 ml)
- 1 teaspoon honey or maple syrup (5 ml)
- ¼ teaspoon black peppercorns (optional)
- 1 bay leaf (optional)

INSTRUCTIONS:

1. Peel the onion and carrot. Thinly slice both and place them in a heat-resistant bowl or glass jar.
2. In a small saucepan, combine the vinegar, water, and honey or maple syrup. Add peppercorns and bay leaf if using.
3. Bring the mixture to a gentle boil, then remove from heat.
4. Pour the hot liquid over the onion and carrot slices, making sure they are fully submerged.
5. Let the slaw cool at room temperature for at least 30 minutes. For deeper flavor, refrigerate and let sit for a few hours or overnight.
6. Serve as a colorful and tangy side or topping for wraps, bowls, or sandwiches.

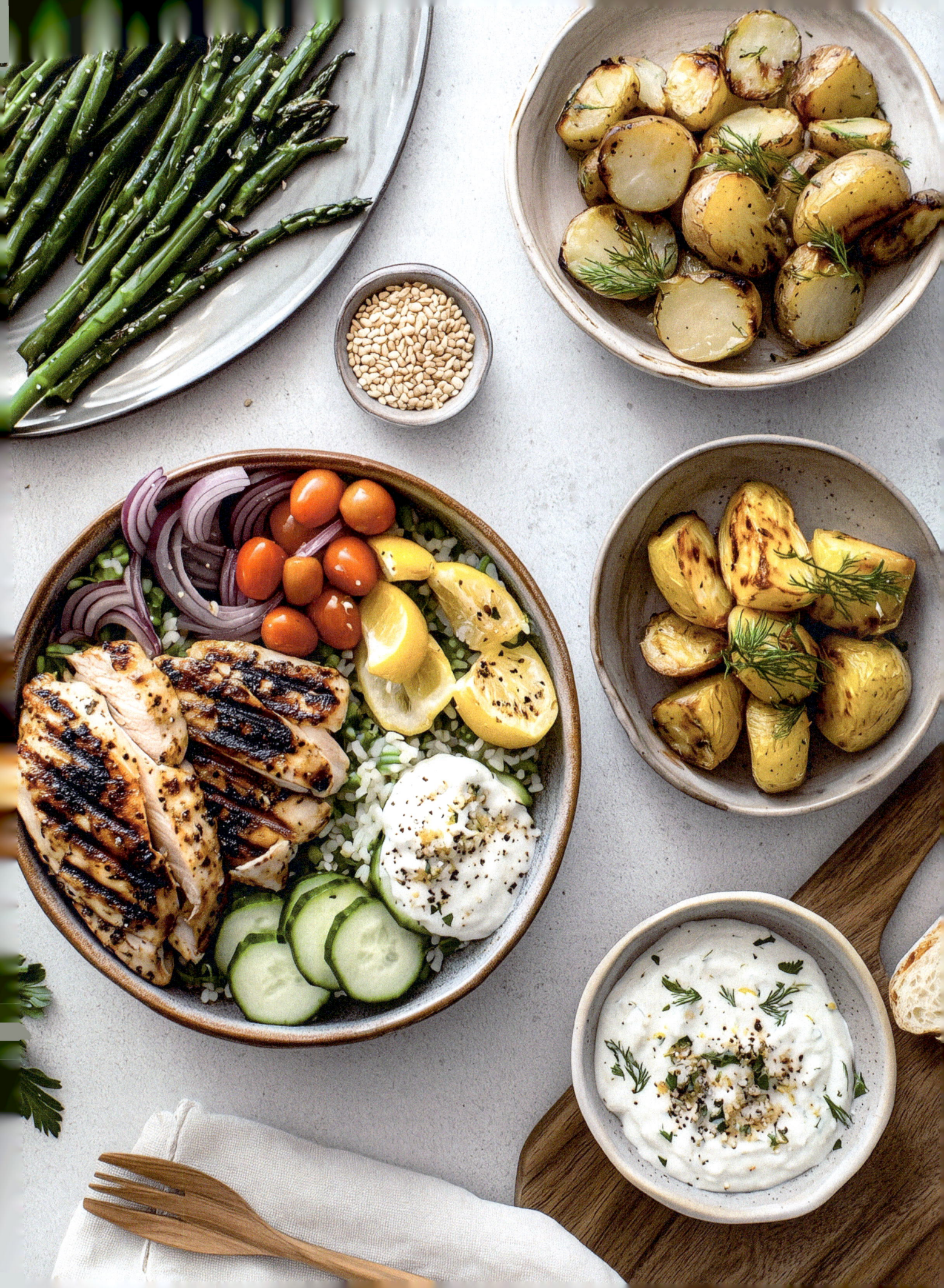

FINAL CHAPTER: YOUR PATH TO LASTING HEALTH

THE MAGIC OF THE DASH DIET

You've done it. Every recipe and change has brought you closer to a healthier, happier version of yourself. Remember, this journey is not about perfection, but about the small decisions that—over time—make a big impact.

And the best part is that you've done it at your own pace, without rushing, enjoying every step.

Eating well doesn't have to be complicated. The DASH diet lets you enjoy delicious foods while caring for your heart and health—without giving up everything you love.

And the best part? You've taken a giant step toward a healthier and more energetic future!

FINAL TIPS FOR LASTING CHANGE

Now that you have the tools and recipes to continue, the most important thing is to make it your own. Here are some practical tips to keep going:

- **Go at your own pace:** You don't need to be perfect. Choose the recipes you enjoy most and adapt them to what you have on hand—or to your lifestyle. The key is consistency. Remember: healthy eating is fun and can fit into your life effortlessly.

- **Stay flexible:** If one day you don't have the ingredients or don't feel like cooking what you planned, that's okay. The DASH diet is flexible. Just choose what works best for you at that moment, always within the principles of the diet. Don't overcomplicate it!

- **Keep exploring new recipes:** Even though you've learned many recipes, there's a whole world of possibilities with DASH. Try new combinations, add fresh ingredients, and enjoy cooking without stress. Healthy cooking is fun, and there's always something new to discover!

WHAT TO DO NOW

Now it's time to take action and make healthy habits part of your daily life.

Here are some practical steps to help you get started:

- **Use the 30-Day Plan:** If you haven't already, check out the 30-Day Plan in Chapter 3. It's designed to help you build a routine, plan your shopping, and organize your meals in a simple, effective way.

- **Adapt the recipes:** You don't have to follow the recipes exactly. If you don't like one or don't have the ingredients, feel free to make changes. The DASH diet is about adapting what works best for you, not being rigid.

- **Remember portion sizes:** Keep in mind the portion recommendations shared in Chapter 2. It's not about being exact, but about knowing how to balance foods on your plate for optimal health.

- **Use your bonus resources:** To support you even further, remember that this book includes three exclusive DASH-friendly bonuses: an exercise guide, special occasion recipes, and a practical DASH toolkit. You'll find the QR code to access them at the beginning of the book. If you haven't downloaded them yet, now is the perfect time to take advantage of these extra tools to make the DASH lifestyle even easier.

STAYING INSPIRED ON YOUR JOURNEY

It's normal sometimes to lose motivation, but here are some resources to keep moving forward:

- **Track your progress:** Record how you feel as you follow the diet. If you notice improvements in your energy, health, or overall well-being, celebrate those small victories. Every step counts.

- **Join a community:** If it helps, look for online groups where you can share your progress or ask questions. It's easier to stay motivated when you have the support of others on the same journey.

- **Be creative and innovative:** Don't be afraid to get creative in the kitchen! You can experiment with new ingredient combinations or even create your own recipes that align with the DASH principles. Sometimes, the best thing is to com-

...good for you.

OF YOUR HEALTH LONG-TERM

The journey to a healthier life doesn't end here. The most important thing is that you've made a great stride. Every step you take brings you closer to a life full of energy and well-being. You don't have to make radical changes; just continue making small adjustments that will help you live better. Remember, if one day you feel demotivated, it's okay. The important thing is to get back on track, adapt it to your life, and continue with confidence. You've earned every small victory, and what's next will be even better.

Thank you for making it this far. Every healthy decision you make is a victory, and I hope you continue enjoying this journey toward a more vibrant life. The path to health begins with the first step, and what awaits you next will be even more rewarding.

YOUR OPINION MATTERS: YOUR REVIEW TRULY MAKE A DIFFERENCE!

Dear Reader,

Thank you for spending time with *The Easy & Tasty DASH Diet Cookbook for Seniors.* I hope the easy-to-follow recipes and heart-friendly ideas in this book have brought flavor and vitality into your kitchen and made healthy eating feel more joyful and sustainable.

Your feedback truly means a lot to me. When you share your thoughts and experiences, you help other seniors make informed choices about improving their diet and health in a realistic, enjoyable way. Reviews can guide new readers by giving them a glimpse of how this cookbook might help them feel more confident in the kitchen and more connected to their well-being.

Your review not only helps others, but also supports my work as an author. It encourages me to keep creating practical and uplifting resources that make healthy eating feel possible and inspiring for everyone. So if this book has made a difference for you—big or small—your review can help that positive impact reach even more people.

With all my thanks,

Amber Hampton

Amber Hampton

JUST SCAN THE QR CODE TO LEAVE YOUR REVIEW.

REFERENCES

American Heart Association. (2023). *DASH Eating Plan.* American Heart Association.

Centers for Disease Control and Prevention. (2022, May 17). *Preventing High Blood Pressure.* Centers for Disease Control and Prevention.

Harvard T.H. Chan School of Public Health. (n.d.). The DASH Diet. https://www.hsph.harvard.edu/nutritionsource/healthy-eating-plate/dash-diet/

Mayo Clinic. (2023). *DASH diet: Healthy eating to lower your blood pressure.* https://www.mayoclinic.org/healthy-lifestyle/nutrition-and-healthy-eating/in-depth/dash-diet/art-20048456

National Heart, Lung, and Blood Institute. (2021). *Your Guide to Lowering Your Blood Pressure with DASH.* https://www.nhlbi.nih.gov/education/dash-eating-plan

National Institutes of Health. (2023). *Dietary Approaches to Stop Hypertension (DASH).* https://www.nhlbi.nih.gov/health/dash-eating-plan

Printed in Dunstable, United Kingdom